T0262825

Pediatric Abdominal Organ Transplantation

Abdominal organ transplantation in children is a complex procedure that requires a multidisciplinary team to ensure that outcomes are consistently excellent. This book highlights the surgical point of view of the surgical aspects of multiorgan transplantation. It is intended to deepen the knowledge of these types of transplants for medical students, nurses, doctors, and anaesthetists. This book will serve to expand the understanding of the general concepts of pediatric abdominal transplantation, focusing on the indications, surgical techniques, and complications of each type of graft for all multidisciplinary team members.

Pediatric Abdominal Organ Transplantation
An Introduction and Practical Guide

Sergio Assia-Zamora and Nigel Heaton

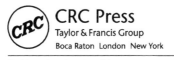

CRC Press
Taylor & Francis Group
Boca Raton London New York

CRC Press is an imprint of the
Taylor & Francis Group, an **Informa** business

Designed cover image: Eduardo González Melgoza

First edition published 2024
by CRC Press
2385 NW Executive Center Drive, Suite 320, Boca Raton, FL 33431

and by CRC Press
4 Park Square, Milton Park, Abingdon, Oxon, OX14 4RN

CRC Press is an imprint of Taylor & Francis Group, LLC

© 2024 Sergio Assia-Zamora and Nigel Heaton

ISBN: 978-1-032-37756-8 (hbk)
ISBN: 978-1-032-37132-0 (pbk)
ISBN: 978-1-003-34174-1 (ebk)

DOI: 10.1201/9781003341741

Typeset in Adobe Garamond Pro
by Apex CoVantage, LLC

Access the Support Material: www.routledge.com/9781032371320

Dedicated to the children who have shaped us into who we are, and to the mentors who have imparted the knowledge that guides us.

Contents

Preface

Transplantation has emerged as a treatment for end-stage organ disease over the last 70 years to transform the lives of patients in a way that was previously considered impossible. The advent of effective immunosuppression led to dramatic improvements in the survival of transplant recipients. Early outcomes have improved to the point that the quality of life and long-term outcomes have become the focus of the multidisciplinary transplant team. The early pioneers focused on the surgeons and the surgical team, however, patients and particularly children have also been pioneers in their own way. The expansion of transplantation particularly over the last 30 years has led to the development of organ shortages and the search for new forms of donation. The rise of living donor transplantation and most recently of machine perfusion to try to improve organ utilization from cadaveric transplantation are the most recent developments.

Today, transplantation requires a multidisciplinary team to provide for consistent high-quality care. This begins with ensuring that there are networks for appropriate referral, assessment at the time of transplantation, and care through to discharge from hospital following successful surgery. With the number of children that have been transplanted, many have reached adulthood with the realization that there is a need for specialist care to nurture these recipients through adolescence and transition into adult long-term follow-up. The focus on nutrition, mental and physical well-being, managing immunosuppression whilst trying to minimize long-term side effects has meant that the multidisciplinary team includes a wide spectrum of specialists providing input and care. This book attempts to provide an understanding of abdominal organ transplantation and the core knowledge that all members of a multidisciplinary team may find helpful.

Looking after children and their families who have faced serious illness and subsequent transplantation, can be a humbling experience. The bravery and fortitude shown by these families in adversity is very powerful. We hope that this book helps to encourage colleagues interested in this field and to provide an understanding of the challenges our children and their families face and how we can provide hope for their future well being.

Sergio Assia-Zamora
Nigel Heaton

Authors

Sergio Assia-Zamora is a pediatrician and pediatric surgeon. Currently, he is Senior Clinical Fellow in Pediatric Liver Transplant at King's College Hospital. He is a member of the following: the European Board of Transplant Surgeons; the European Board of Pediatric Surgeons; American Society of Transplant Surgeons; British Association of Pediatric Surgeons; Royal College of Surgeons Liver Transplant; Royal College of Surgeons; International Liver Transplant Society; British Transplant Society; Pediatric Surgical Council; Pediatric Council; and the Mexican Society of Transplantation. His special interests are within pediatric transplantation and complex renal and hepatobiliary surgery as well as auxiliary liver transplant. His research interests include liver regeneration, 3D printing models, machine perfusion and pathologies related to ductal plate malformations.

Nigel Heaton is Head of Liver Transplantation at King's College Hospital NHSFT and was previously the Clinical Academic Co-Lead for Liver, Renal, Urology, GI Medicine and Surgery and Transplantation within King's Health Partners, the Academic Health Centre serving South London. He is an adult and pediatric liver transplant and HPB surgeon, and has been responsible for the Liver Transplant Programme at King's College Hospital for the past 20+ years. The unit performs over 240 transplants per year in adults and children. In the last 25 years, the unit has performed more than 6,000 liver transplants including over 1,200 in children. The unit also has programmes for pediatric small bowel and multi-visceral transplantation and islet and hepatocyte cell therapy. His specific interests within liver transplant surgery include split and auxiliary liver transplantation and liver regeneration. His research interests include liver regeneration, ischemia reperfusion injury, and primary liver cancer.

Contributors

Anna Adamusiak, MD, PhD, FEBS
Specialty Doctor in Pediatric Renal
    Transplantation
Guy's and St. Thomas' NHS
    Foundation Trust, UK

Rob Broomhead, MBCHB, DCH,
    FRCA
Anaesthetic Consultant Liver Transplant
King's College Hospital
and
Anaesthetic Consultant
Cleveland Clinic, UK

Miriam Cortés-Cerisuelo, MD, PhD
Liver Transplant Surgeon Consultant
King's College Hospital, UK

Anil Dhawan, MD, FRCPCH
Director Research and Innovation
Pediatric Liver, GI and Nutrition
    Centre and Mowat Labs
King's College Hospital, UK

Andrea Fernandez-Pujol, MD
Senior Clinical Fellow
Hepatobiliary Surgery
and
Consultant General Surgeon
King's College Hospital, UK

Sahil Gupta, MBBS, MS, MCh
Senior Clinical Fellow
Hepatobiliary and Liver Transplant
    Surgery
King's College Hospital, UK

Wayel Jassem, MD, PhD
Liver Transplant Surgeon Consultant
King's College Hospital, UK

Lianne Miller
Liver Theatre Clinical Coordinator
Kings College Hospital, UK

Buddhika Uragoda-Appuhamilage
Clinical Fellow in Transplant
    Surgery
King's College Hospital, UK

Anita Verma
Infectologist
Pediatric Liver, GI and Nutrition
    Centre and Mowat Labs
King's College Hospital, UK

Hector Vilca-Melendez,
    MD, PhD
Liver Transplant Surgeon
    Consultant
King's College Hospital, UK

Sunitha Vimalesvaran, MBBS,
    MRCPCH
Pediatric Hepatology Registrar
Pediatric Liver, GI and Nutrition
    Centre and Mowat Labs
King's College Hospital, UK

Melinda Yii
Senior Sister
Liver Theatre Clinical Coordinator
King's College Hospital, UK

Drawings by:

Eduardo González Melgoza
Software Engineer, Tech
    Mahindra
Professor, Tecnológico de Monterrey
Freelance Digital Artist, Mexico

1 Introduction

Transplantation has become the accepted treatment for children with end-stage organ disease. Transplantation is associated with longer survival, improved growth, neurodevelopment, cognitive function, and overall quality of life (QOL).

Abdominal organ transplantation in children is a complex procedure which requires multidisciplinary teams working together in specialised centers. Experienced pediatricians, anesthetics, and surgeons working closely with nursing, dietetic, physiotherapy, transplant co-ordinators, psychologists, play therapists and pharmacy teams to assess, transplant and follow-up children through this journey.

Transplant surgery of all organs demands the technical ability to perform complex vascular anastomoses to join vessels, bile ducts, ureters or bowel without a leak, stricture, or clot formation. Tissue matching for donor and recipient is important for some organs such as the kidney and less so for others like the liver. Matching for blood group ia important. However, it was the introduction of effective immunosuppression in the form of cyclosporine which transformed the specialty from pioneering to a established clinical service in the early 1980s. There are several immunosuppression protocols, but all are based around calcineurin inhibitors including cyclosporine and Tacrolimus. More recently it has been possible to transplant across blood type by physically removing Antibodies from the blood in combination with specialized immunosuppressive protocols.

Currently organ shortage is the limiting factor in restricting transplant activity. The development of living donation has been important for increasing liver and kidney transplantation worldwide. This in turn is driving interest in laparoscopic and robotic surgical techniques to encourage living donation. In addition, this raised interest in the ethics of donation and the international regulation of transplant activity particularly about organ trafficking and donor safety. Most recently the introduction of machine perfusion especially in liver transplantation has opened a new chapter in transplant history. With this success there has been a huge growth in the numbers of recipients being followed up and a focus on long-term outcomes and particularly the quality of life. There remain significant challenges, not least the inequalities of access to medical care and transplantation that exist worldwide.

This book is organized in chapters on each abdominal organ separately starting with kidney transplantation which is the most commonly performed transplant worldwide.

DOI: 10.1201/9781003341741-1

2 History of abdominal organ transplantation

In the twentieth century, the idea of organ transplantation evolved into a medical treatment, despite facing numerous challenges along the way. Advancements in surgical, anesthetic and intensive care enabled pioneering surgeons to perform organ transplants successfully. However, other challenges had to be overcome including understanding of the immune system and tissue rejection, organ preservation and the management of immunosuppression and infection.

There is a wealth of literature about the history of transplantation, including scientific publications, biographies of transplant pioneers and recipients and the world's press. This chapter aims to present a chronological account of their work, which has led to the current state of pediatric organ transplantation.

2.1 RENAL TRANSPLANTATION

The concept of re-establishing the blood flow to the implanted organ is made possible through connecting blood vessels. Vascular anastomosis is paramount for restoring arterial in-flow and venous out-flow to allow the transplanted kidney to function. Pioneering work in kidney transplantation paralleled the development of vascular surgery techniques. In 1877, Nikolai Eck used silk stitches to join the portal vein and vena cava to create a portosystemic shunt and treat portal hypertension. John Benjamin Murphy achieved the very first successful connection of two ends of an artery in clinical practice in 1897 in Chicago, to repair a gunshot injury of the femoral artery.

In the early 1900s, Alexis Carrel in Lyon and Erwin Payr in Vienna pioneered vascular anastomosis techniques that enabled experimental kidney transplantation be performed. In 1901, Payr introduced a device derived from the elaboration of the standard method for rubber tubing connection. It was based on the external ligature of vascular stumps over an absorbable magnesium ring. Robert Abbe in New York first reported using the inner hollow tubes for connecting blood vessels in 1894, and developed vascular stents made out of glass.

In 1896 Mathieu Jaboulay, the head of the Surgery Department in Lyon, was the first to publish good results from suturing blood vessels in animal experiments – he used the technique of interrupted sutures. Alexis Carrel was aware of this work, but developed a different technique. He developed the method of suturing

DOI: 10.1201/9781003341741-2

blood vessels was performed with end to end with support threads (so-called stay sutures) in a triangular fashion, thus holding the vessel open and keeping the back wall clear of the stitching in the front. What undoubtedly contributed to Carrel's outcomes that outdistanced those of his peers were thinner needles and finer suture material he used and the meticulous suturing skills he learned during sewing lessons from a French embroiderer.

In 1902, Emerich Ullmann in Vienna reported evidence of a functioning renal auto transplant implanted in a dog's neck. He used Payr's stenting technique to connect the blood vessels. That same year, also in Vienna, Alfred von Decastello performed dog-to-dog kidney transplantation. Ullmann subsequently carried out renal xenotransplantation (cross-species transplant) putting a dog's kidney into a goat's neck and a pig's kidney into the elbow of a young woman with end-stage renal disease. Although both Ullman and von Decastello abandoned further research in kidney transplantation, many European surgeons developed an interest in the field and carried out further animal experiments. In 1905, Nicholas Floresco in Bucharest reported two modifications to the experimental kidney transplant technique. He connected the ureter to the bladder instead of leading onto the surface of the skin as his predecessors had done and also flushed out the blood from the donor's kidney with normal saline prior to the orthotropic implantation in the correct anatomical position (orthotopic).

Carrel subsequently left France and relocated to the United States, where he collaborated with American surgeon Charles Guthrie in Chicago from 1905 to 1906. Subsequently, he became the head of experimental surgery at the Rockefeller Institute for Medical Research in New York. During this time, he made further advancements to the vascular anastomosis technique and conducted experiments on animals.

Together with Guthrie, Carrel developed a technique for dealing with small vessels, where the donor artery is not directly stitched but remains attached to a sizable cut from its larger vessel of origin. They demonstrated the feasibility of preserving arteries in cold storage for over 20 hours before implanting them and showed that a vein patch could be used to replace a segment of the artery.

In recognition of his groundbreaking work in organ transplantation, Alexis Carrel was awarded the Nobel Prize in 1912.

During the early 1900s, surgeons in Europe and the United States made significant progress in demonstrating the technical feasibility of vascular anastomosis (connecting blood vessels) for organ transplantation. They performed various experiments on animals to study the transplantation of organs from one individual to another.

It was not until later in the twentieth century, with greater understanding of immunology and particularly the discovery of acquired immunological tolerance by Peter Medawar and Sir Macfarlane Burnet. Their work on rejection and tolerance of skin grafts which led to them sharing the Nobel Prize in Medicine in 1960. Medawar later was regarded as the 'father of transplantation. However, it was the development of effective immunosuppressive drugs, that allowed successful organ transplantation to be performed between different individuals of the same species. The introduction of cyclosporin by Sir Roy Calne produced a dramatic change in outcome and the beginning of the acceptance of transplantation into mainstream medicine. These breakthroughs paved the way for modern organ transplantation, saving countless lives and improving the quality of life for many patients with organ failure.

In 1906, Mathieu Jaboulay conducted two kidney transplants on patients suffering from chronic renal failure. He used a pig and a goat as donors and implanted the organs in the patients' arm and thigh, respectively. Although the transplants produced urine for 3 days, they eventually failed due to thrombosis.

In 1909, Ernst Unger attempted to transplant kidneys from a 10-year-old pig-tailed macaque into a young woman with renal failure. He performed a simultaneous surgery, connecting the donor's vena cava and aorta to the recipient's femoral vessels in the upper thigh of the recipient. However, the transplanted kidneys did not produce urine, and the patient passed away within 2 days of the surgery.

During that era, the use of animals as donors for transplantation was considered acceptable because there were reports of successful grafting of animal tissues like corneas and bones in the surgical literature. Moreover, since dialysis had not yet been developed, patients with kidney failure had no effective form of kidney support and died. The lack of understanding of how the immune system functioned led to attempts at human xenotransplantation which in hindsight seem primitive and unsurprisingly failed and subsequently abandoned until very recent times.

In 1933, a Ukrainian surgeon Yurii Voronoy performed the first human-to-human kidney transplant. At that time, it was recognized that when the kidney remained without a blood supply (warm ischemia) outside the body that it impacted on its subsequent function, leading to efforts to minimize this time. The kidney needed to be recovered from the recently deceased donor immediately, followed by recipient surgery, which presented logistical challenges.

In the Soviet Union, obtaining tissue from deceased donors was possible without significant legal formalities, and procuring blood from fresh cadavers was already practiced. Deceased donors were also a source of corneal grafts.

In this particular case, Voronoy recovered the kidney from a 60-year-old man who had suffered a head injury and died upon arrival at the hospital. The recipient was a 26-year-old woman who had been anuric for 4 days after attempting suicide by ingesting mercuric chloride. The blood groups of the donor and recipient were different, with the donor being blood group B and the recipient being blood group O. The kidney was joined to blood vessels in the thigh and appeared to work for a short time before the blood vessels thrombosed (from rejection) and the patient subsequently died.

In the late 1940s, interest in experimental transplantation was stimulated by increasing knowledge of the immune system and research into skin grafting, leading to further attempts at human allotransplantation. Pioneering human allotransplants in the early 1950s were performed with limited. Immunosuppression using steroids.

In 1950, Richard Lawler performed a kidney transplant on a 44-year-old woman with renal polycystic disease. He used a blood type-matched deceased donor kidney, implanting it after removing the patient's polycystic kidney during the same procedure. The transplant initially functioned well, but later encountered issues. Lawler's effort sparked public interest in renal transplantation. In France, three teams performed nine kidney transplants in the early 1950s, with the first two using kidneys from a guillotined prisoner. Unfortunately, these kidneys did not function satisfactorily after transplantation.

In 1952, the first kidney transplant using a relative's donated organ was performed in Paris on a 16-year-old carpenter. The kidney from his mother initially worked well, but it abruptly failed after 22 days, and the patient died. Around this time, surgeons in Boston used a prototype dialysis machine to support patients after kidney transplant until the donor kidney began to function. In 1951, David Hume initiated human kidney transplants, and his patients were the first to undergo pre-surgery dialysis. In 1947, Hume and his colleagues performed a successful bedside kidney transplant, but details were only publicized years later.

Between 1951 and 1953, David Hume conducted nine kidney transplants. The donor kidneys were obtained from patients who died during heart surgery or children who underwent the Matson procedure. Out of the nine transplants, five failed to function at all, while the other four showed some function for several weeks to several months.

In December 1954, Joseph Murray took over at Brigham Hospital and performed a successful kidney transplant between identical twins thereby avoiding problems with rejection. This demonstrated that matching recipients with genetically identical donors could prevent rejection and allow for long-term graft function. The kidney was placed in the pelvis, and the patient recovered well. This success led to further twin transplants, totalling 29 pairs by 1976.

The development of immunosuppression protocols in the following decade transformed kidney transplantation from a challenging procedure confined to academic centers in developed countries into a routine service available worldwide for patients with renal failure.

As of 2021, the number of pediatric candidates waiting for kidney transplants continues to rise, with 1,087 added to the waiting list that year. Candidates aged 12 years and older constituted the largest proportion at 67.3%. The total number of pediatric kidney transplants performed also reached its highest point in a decade, with 820 transplants in 2021. Living donor kidney transplants accounted for 28.5% of total transplants among pediatric recipients that year.

In 2021, 36 programs were exclusively performing pediatric kidney transplants, while 136 were focused on adult transplants, and 54 handled transplants for both adults and children.

2.2 TRANSPLANT IMMUNOLOGY

In 1910, the Nobel Prize was awarded to Paul Ehrlich and Elie Metchnikoff for their research on the human body's immunological response to microorganisms. Ehrlich demonstrated antibodies neutralizing bacterial toxins, while Metchnikoff showed the involvement of phagocytes in this response. However, the immunological mechanism behind graft failure was not considered at that time.

Transplantation immunology's origin is credited to Georg Schone, a German surgeon, who experimented with tumour transplantation in animals in the nineteenth century. He found that grafts failed more rapidly when transplanted into genetically different animals. Schone's work suggested that allografts were lost due to the recipient's immune system response to the donor tissue.

During World War II, improving outcomes of skin grafts for burns became a focus. Tom Gibson and Peter Medawar proposed an immunological mechanism for graft loss in allotransplantation. This paradigm of immune response leading to rejection was accepted by the scientific community.

In 1948, cortisone was first used to treat rheumatoid arthritis, showing some immunosuppressive effects in experimental transplantation. In the early 1950s, Medawar reported graft acceptance in animals after pre-treatment with irradiation and bone marrow infusion. However, graft-versus-host disease caused serious complication in clinical practice. Sublethal irradiation alone proved to be immunosuppressive, achieving long-term survival in kidney recipients.

In 1958, attempts at human bone marrow transplantation used irradiation for pre-conditioning, but poor results led to the exploration of anti-cancer drugs such as 6-mercaptopurine (6-MP) for immunosuppression. Roy Calne found 6-MP to be effective in prolonging kidney allograft survival in dogs. Subsequently Azathioprine, a derivative of 6-MP, became available for human use in 1961, and its combination with prednisolone became a standard regimen in kidney transplantation.

In the 1980s, cyclosporine became the dominant immunosuppressive agent, followed by the introduction of newer drugs like tacrolimus, mycophenolate mofetil, and rapamycin in the 1990s. Ongoing efforts aim to optimize and tailor immunosuppression regimens, with the development of modern agents, including monoclonal antibodies targeting specific immunological responses in transplanted organs.

2.3 LIVER TRANSPLANTATION

In 1955, Stewart Welch reported the first experimental liver transplant in dogs at Albany Medical College, using an axillary hepatic allograft. In 1958, Francis Moore described an orthotopic liver transplant in Boston.

Thomas Starzl attempted the first human liver transplants after the success of azathioprine and steroid immunosuppression in kidney transplantation. He performed several experimental liver transplants in dogs with varying methods of restoring portal flow, with some surviving for up to 3 weeks.

Starzl conducted the first human liver transplant in 1965 on a 3-year-old boy with biliary atresia. Unfortunately, the patient did not survive due to massive blood loss during surgery. Other early attempts by Starzl, Moore, and Jean Demirleau in Paris also had disappointing outcomes.

Starzl temporarily halted his liver transplant program and developed procedures and principles to guide liver transplantation. He resumed the program in 1967, adding anti-thymocyte globulin to the immunosuppression regime. Eight subsequent pedlatric patients survived the surgery with four of them died from sepsis within a few months.

In 1998, Roy Calne performed the first liver transplant attempt on a child in Cambridge, UK, but the recipient with biliary atresia died during the surgery.

After establishing liver transplantation in Denver, Starzl moved his program to Pittsburgh in 1981, transplanting a further 808 children up to 1998. Prior to the introduction of cyclosporin infectious complications, bile leak and acute and chronic rejection were responsible for the high early mortality which in the 1970s was as high as 70%-80%. At one year! In 1968, Roy Calne performed the first liver transplant in Cambridge, UK. Calne introduced cyclosporine in in 1979 which by 1982 had transformed the landscape of transplantation forever. Starzl subsequently reported the use of Tacrolimus in 1990 which has become the most widely used immunosuppressant in transplantation.

The shortage of size-matched cadaveric liver donors for children drove technical innovation utilizing knowledge of the segmental anatomy of the liver. This allowed for a larger liver to be used to transplant a smaller recipient. The ex situ liver reduction technique, described by Henri Bismuth in 1984, became standard practice in children and was further refined to liver splitting to benefit two recipients from one liver by Rudolf Pichylmayer in 1988. Splitting evolved so that it could be performed ex-situ on the back table or in situ in heart-beating cadaveric donor, in an identical technique to procuring a left lateral segment from a living donor.

2.4 PANCREAS TRANSPLANTATION

In 1966, William Kelly and Richard Lillehei at the University of Minnesota performed the first vascularized human cadaveric pancreatic transplant on a 28-year-old woman with diabetes and end-stage renal disease. They transplanted a segment of the pancreas tail which functioned for over 2 month, in conjunction with a kidney from the same donor.

David Sutherland, who worked at the University of Minnesota from the 1970s until 2010, performed numerous pancreas transplants, refining surgical techniques and management over time. Edison Teixeira performed the first isolated segmental pancreatic transplant in 1966. In 1979, Sutherland performed the first living related transplantation of the pancreatic tail and pioneered protocols for isolating and infusing pancreatic islets. The introduction of Tacrolimus and mycophenolate mofetil in the early 1990s led to significant improvement in outcomes and increased numbers of transplants.

Pancreas transplantation in children is rare. Some cases involve simultaneous kidney and pancreas transplants in teenagers with type 1 diabetes and diabetic nephropathy. In selected cases where benefits outweigh the risks, pancreas transplant alone can be considered for patients not needing a kidney transplant. The youngest known recipient of an isolated pancreas transplant alone was 11 years old, but graft function was lost within 6 months. In 2018, a 13-year-old girl with an insulin allergy received a pancreas transplant at the University of Minnesota, which continues to function 5 years later.

2.5 INTESTINAL TRANSPLANTATION

The early clinical attempts at human intestinal transplantation were made in Boston in 1964 on two children, with their mothers as donors. Unfortunately, both attempts failed, and the children died.

In March 1967, Richard Lillehei at the University of Minnesota performed the first adult intestinal transplant on a 46-year-old woman with short gut due to massive mesenteric vein thrombosis and extensive bowel resection. The transplant involved the whole small bowel taken from a brain-dead donor. While the immediate postoperative period seemed promising with adequate blood flow and peristalsis, the patient died several hours after the operation due to extensive portal vein thrombosis and caval thrombosis resulting in graft infarction. Lillehei also attempted a triple transplantation in July 1967, involving intestine, pancreas, and kidney, but the recipient only survived for one month. Subsequent attempts worldwide did not achieve long-term success, and the field paused until the era of Cyclosporin.

In 1971, researchers reported that intestinal grafts were often associated with graft-versus-host disease (GVHD), leading to destruction of the host organs by immunocompetent cells from the donor graft. GVHD has been frequently observed in clinical intestinal transplantation and the balance between infection, rejection and GVHD is a fine one.

The practice of intestinal transplantation was rekindled in Toronto in 1985, using bowel segments from living-related donors. In around 1988, a new strategy involving the en-bloc procedure gained popularity. This approach included transplanting the liver, and possibly the pancreas and stomach, along with the intestines. The first successful report with this technique came from David Grant in London, Ontario. The en-bloc strategy was technically attractive and found support from observations that the liver provided protective immunological effect on simultaneous grafts. In 1988, Starzl attempted various anatomical strategies for multivisceral transplants and reported a 75% 1-year survival rate when using tacrolimus. Intestinal and multivisceral transplantation was established in Pittsburg and has been taken up by many centers internationally.

3

Organ donation and retrieval

The donor operation is an integral part of the transplantation process. A well-executed multiorgan recovery is essential for a successful implant. Operating on living donors requires technical mastery and additional considerations to minimise the burden of surgery since this group of patients does not directly benefit from the procedure.

Donation can only take place if legal requirements of it are fulfilled. A living donor needs to sign an informed consent. Requirements for obtaining organs from deceased donors differ between countries. In the opt-in model, permission is usually obtained from the next of kin, aware of the potential donor's wishes. In the opt-out model, it needs to be verified if a potential donor specifically expressed unwillingness to donate.

The deceased donation can happen either after death diagnosed by brainstem function test – donors after brainstem death (DBD) – or death diagnosed by cessation of the effective circulation – donors after circulatory death (DCD).

The donation process requires excluding the presence of contraindications and assessment of the suitability of organs in order to allocate them to adequate recipients. Once the potential donor has been identified, the donor coordinator records all relevant information and maintains open communication with the recipient teams.

Experienced surgeons should perform the retrieval operation with adequate assistance due to the complexity and the challenging anatomical variations that can be encountered. Sometimes, the donors might not have had sufficient or any abdominal imaging. The surgical procedure should be harmonic between the cardiothoracic team involved and the abdominal team, maintaining clear communication and synchronic movements to perform a successful retrieval, especially when it is a multiorgan retrieval.

In many countries, living donation is the only transplant option, requiring careful evaluation of the donor, anatomical variations, and comorbidities to minimize operative morbidity and mortality and facilitate the best results for the recipient without jeopardizing the donor.

The donor surgeon is responsible for the whole retrieval team. They need to review the donor information, including the brainstem death test in DBD donors, consent for donation, blood tests, and the circumstances of death.

DOI: 10.1201/9781003341741-3

At the time of retrieval, the anatomy, organ quality, and findings should be determined to guide the optimal use of the organs. Brains stem death test in DBD donors, consent for donation, blood tests, and the circumstances of death.

3.1 DECEASED ORGAN DONATION

In pediatrics, most transplants are performed with DBD donor grafts worldwide. In recent years, deceased donors have increased considering DCD grafts, hence, the importance of adequate and careful donor selection and evaluation.

There are important differences in the retrieval operation between DBD and DCD donors. In general terms, the DBD procedure consists of two phases, the warm phase and the cold phase, whereas the DCD procedure involves rapid cannulation of the aorta, and the whole surgery takes place in the cold phase.

The anatomy during the retrieval is found at its best, especially when it is a DBD donor, since the organs in situ, vessels pulsate, and structures can be identified. In case there is aberrant anatomy, this implies another challenge especially in the second part of the retrieval, or the cold phase.

During the retrieval operation, in DBD donors, during the warm phase, the findings must be verbalized and recorded in order for the recipient centers to be informed. The trans-operative assessment technique includes an evaluation and aspect of the organs, including color, shape, and consistency. The liver and pancreas should be assessed on the degree of steatosis and kidneys on their size as well as small bowel.

After the warm phase has been performed and the donor is prepared for the cross clamp and cold phase, the organs must be prepared for a safe extraction, minimizing the risk of damaging of any structures and optimizing the perfusion with preservation fluid. When the recipient centers and donor teams are ready for cross clamp, aortic cannulation should be unequivocal for optimization of administration of the perfusion fluid.

With cold preservation solution through the main vessels, namely aorta, and portal vein for the liver, the organs must appear soft, cold, and uniformly perfused with no areas of congestion.

In the case of DCD donors, there is only a cold phase and dissection is performed only with cold cutting, always guaranteeing adequate perfusion of the abdominal organs in order to minimize the risk of delayed or primary graft nonfunction. Organs retrieved from DCD donors, are subject to warm ischemia during the agonal phase, especially in liver and pancreas. The utilization of these organs has progressed with caution and results are still being analyzed.

In the case of living donation, the risks to the donor are well recognized, and the assessment of any potential donor is essential to ensure appropriate donor and recipient selection. Living donation should only be performed if the risk to the donor is justified by the expectation of an acceptable outcome for the recipient.

Recently, there has been growing technical expertise in the living donor operation, anatomical variations are better assessed and dealt with, in order to provide the best quality organs for the recipients. In case of living donor liver transplant, optimal assessment and evaluation and operation techniques reduce the incidence of small-for-size syndrome for the recipient despite sometimes having a higher risk of technical complications.

3.2 CONTRAINDICATIONS TO DONATION

The contraindications to donation are dynamic given the increasing experience and knowledge about the risks posed to the recipient according to the donor history. The donor team must keep all of this in mind and obtain as much information from the donor as possible as well as accurate details of the surgical operation for the right decisions to be made.

3.3 RETRIEVAL OPERATION

A midline incision is carefully made, running from the sternal notch to the pubic symphysis, to access the abdominal cavity. A laparotomy is then performed, and the falciform ligament is carefully detached up to the level of the hepatic veins. At this point, the surgeon inspects the abdominal organs, visually assessing and palpating them to rule out any malignancies or unexpected findings, such as pancreatitis. These findings should be kept in mind during the subsequent dissection of the hilium.

The suprasternal notch is dissected, with caution taken not to damage the great veins, as this could result in significant bleeding. The surgeon creates a tunnel using their left index finger and creates a lower tunnel bluntly using their right index finger under the xiphoid process. Next, the long Debakey forceps are passed, and a Gigli saw is used to carefully open the sternum from top to bottom. During this step, the operating table may be adjusted depending on the surgeon's height, and the lungs may be temporarily deflated if approved by the anaesthesia team. An alternative is to use an electric sternotomy device.

The chest is opened carefully to avoid damage to vital structures, and the surface of the liver is protected with a swab to prevent injuries. Any adhesions to the liver are carefully divided to avoid damage during the cold phase of the procedure. Bleeding from either side of the cut end of the bone is common but can be easily controlled with bone wax or by applying folded gauze and using a small Finochietto retractor. During the retraction, the surgeon may encounter resistance, which can be relieved somewhat by cutting the diagrammatic fibres from the abdominal side. However, it is important to exercise caution and avoid making holes in the diaphragm during this maneuver, especially if cardiac block anaesthesia is an option.

Following this, a complete Cattell-Braasch maneuver (Figure 3.1) is performed to expose the abdominal aorta, and the duodenum is kocherised to reveal the left renal vein and the intrahepatic inferior vena cava. Before proceeding with this step, it is essential to isolate the small bowel in a single pack to facilitate its retraction by the assistant, particularly in obese patients. Throughout the dissection, the assistance of an experienced assistant is crucial in guiding the tissue plane by using their left index finger.

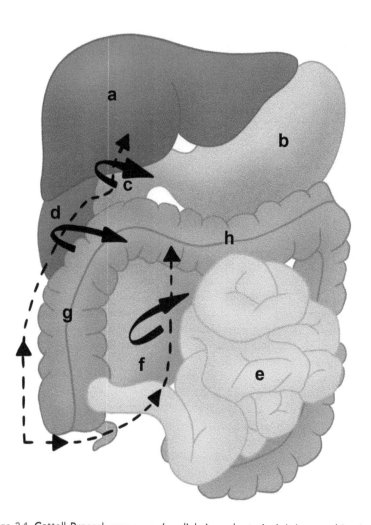

Figure 3.1 **Cattell-Braasch maneuver (medial visceral rotation).** It is a combination of right colonic mobilization and duodenal kocherization, with the dotted line showing the line of dissection. This step is performed at the beginning of the donor surgery to expose the aorta and the left renal vein. One should be very careful not to strip or use diathermy near the right ureter, especially in thin patients where the tissue plane might be easily missed. During pancreas retrieval, the assistant should handle the duodenum very gently to avoid causing a hematoma on the undersurface of the pancreas.

*** a – liver, b – stomach, c – duodenum, d – right kidney, e – small bowel, f – mesentery, g – ascending colon, h – transverse colon.

The entire process requires precision, skill, and meticulous attention to detail to ensure a successful and safe surgical procedure. The collaboration between the surgical team members and their careful handling of the donor anatomy play an important role in the graft functions as well as possible in the recipient.

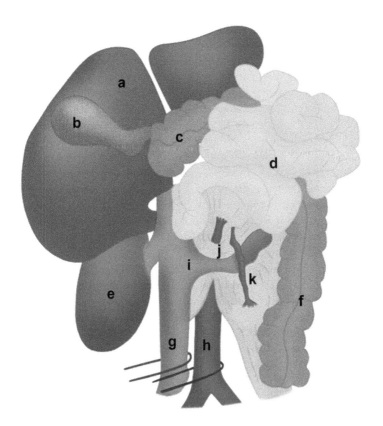

Figure 3.2 Looping of the aorta and preparation for cannulation after Cattell-Braasch maneuver. Note the location of the aorta between IMV and the DJ flexure in case of rapid access to aorta without Cattell-Braasch maneuver.

*** a – liver, b – gallbladder, c – pancreas, d – small bowel, e – right kidney, f – descending colon, g – vena cava, h – aorta, i – left hepatic vein, j – superior mesenteric artery, k – inferior mesenteric vein.

The left triangular ligament is then divided to allow exposure of the hepatogastric ligament. During this step, it is important to place a folded gauze towel under the left lateral segment of the liver to protect the stomach from the diathermy injury. Care should be taken not to damage the left hepatic vein at the medial end of the triangular ligament.

Afterwards, the lesser sac is opened to check for the presence of aberrant arterial anatomy and to inspect the pancreas. This is the moment when a left accessory or replaced left hepatic artery is identified. In the hepato-duodenal ligament, a right accessory or replaced right hepatic artery arising from the superior mesenteric artery and is usually found behind the common bile duct.

Next, the aorta can be looped (Figure 3.2). This step can be performed earlier in the surgery if the donor is unstable and the situation requires rapid cannulation. A landmark for this is between the plane of the DJ flexure and the inferior mesenteric artery, which directly goes into the aorta. In other situations, especially in patients with more visceral fat, one can identify the level and position of the aorta by palpating the pelvis up to the sacral promontory, where the bifurcation is easily felt. The level of dissection is usually longitudinal, following the line of the aorta, and ensuring not to strip the ureter. Once the aorta is identified, it is important to dissect on either side of the aorta, being careful not to damage the lumbar vessels, which can lead to torrential bleeding. Right-angle forceps should be passed under the aorta from medial to lateral to protect the inferior vena cava (IVC) without exerting undue resistance, especially in donors with severe atherosclerosis. After passing three loops around the aorta, it can be mounted on the mosquito forceps. If the aorta is fragile and dilated, it is advisable to use nylon tapes instead of 2.0 silk. In cases where the lower polar renal artery is visible, the area of cannulation can be brought down to the iliac region.

The common bile duct is then dissected and divided above the duodenum, ligating the distal end. The gallbladder can be flushed at this point or during the cold phase. The amount of hilar dissection in the warm phase varies from a no-touch technique to a complete dissection of the hepatic artery and depends on a case-by-case basis by the lead retrieval surgeon.

The dissection target would be to isolate the gastroduodenal artery (GDA) and the splenic artery. Anatomical variations of the hepatic artery should be kept in mind, specifically the low division of the hepatic artery, which can be easily misidentified as the GDA, particularly when the pancreas is also being considered for retrieval. Therefore, it is advisable to clear the junction of the hepatic artery and GDA to avoid misidentifications. However, one should be very careful not to create unnecessary hematoma on the pancreas, which could prevent it from being used.

The location of the accessory right hepatic artery (RHA) is usually posterior and lateral to the portal vein (PV). Once identified, it should be traced down to the superior mesenteric artery (SMA) if the pancreas is not being considered for retrieval. However, if the pancreas is included, the retrieval surgeon should contact both the liver and pancreas recipient centers and come to an agreement to cut the accessory RHA at a level where it can be connected to the GDA stump.

If the pancreas is being considered for retrieval, it is beneficial to isolate the portal vein to start portal venous (PV) perfusion above the pancreas. However, if the pancreas is not on offer, the superior mesenteric vein (SMV) can be cannulated below the pancreas, and the cannula can be directed towards the PV.

At this point, the retrieval surgeon should determine the level of the cross-clamping. It can be done in the abdomen at the supra celiac aorta or at the descending aorta in the chest. If it is done in the abdomen, it is important to isolate and prepare it for cross-clamping by dividing the crus fibres (Figure 3.3). Another option is to use a double balloon to cross clamp.

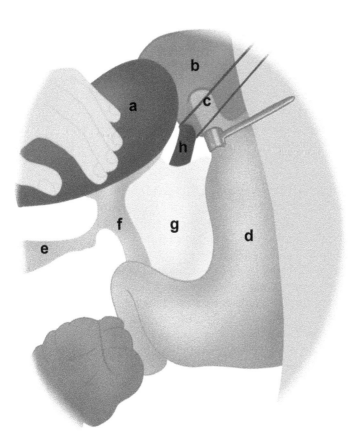

Figure 3.3 Isolation of the supra celiac aorta for cross-clamping in the abdomen. Note that the stomach is retracted laterally by the assistant to expose the right crus over the aorta while the left lobe of the liver is retracted by the surgeon.

*** a – liver, b – diaphragm, c – oesophagus, d – stomach, e – gallbladder, f – common bile duct in hepatic porta, g – gastro-hepatic ligament, h – aorta.

Venting can be done 3 to 5 minutes after the administration of heparin (300–500 IU/kg), in the supra-diaphragmatic region or in the abdomen. If the cardiac block is not an option, it is always preferred to do venting in the chest to avoid pooling blood in the abdomen, which could make the cold phase dissection more difficult.

The abdominal aorta, located below the Inferior Mesenteric Artery (IMA) and before the bifurcation of the iliac arteries between the loops, is identified for cannulation. First, the bottom aorta is tied off. At this point, the surgeon should inform the anaesthetist of the possibility of a sudden increase in blood pressure. Then, the aorta is pressed against the vertebra by the left hand of the surgeon, leaving some space with the bottom tie. Subsequently, a small incision is made in the aorta for cannulation. One should ensure not to insert the cannula too high to prevent poor perfusion of the kidneys. The assistant then places two ties, and all three are tied together. The surgeon can proceed with the venting and the cross-clamping and the time is marked. The abdominal cavity is then filled with crushed ice for rapid cooling of the organs.

The hilar structures are then identified in the cold phase and the dissection starts by dividing the previously identified gastroduodenal artery and the pancreatic end is marked with a prolene suture for the identification during the pancreatic bench surgery.

The left renal vein is divided at the origin of the IVC and the infrahepatic IVC is divided to drain the renal venous blood. The portal vein is divided next, 1 cm above the confluence between the splenic vein and superior mesenteric vein to allow adequate implantation of the pancreas.

The common hepatic artery is dissected towards the celiac axis. The origin of the splenic artery is identified and divided; the distal splenic end of the splenic artery is also marked with a suture for identification during pancreatic bench surgery.

The celiac axis is then dissected from the surrounding lymphatic tissue with a patch of aorta. The diaphragm is then divided around the suprahepatic cava, starting on the left side of the vena cava, continuing posteriorly and completing the division by taking a patch of the right hemidiaphragm around the right lobe of the liver. Dissection is assisted by inserting a finger in the supra-hepatic IVC. The right lobe is separated from the right adrenal gland and the right kidney, the retroperitoneal tissue at the back of the IVC and aorta is divided and the liver is removed and placed in cold preservation solution on ice.

The pancreas is the next organ to be retrieved and a stapler is applied prepyloric dividing the stomach before the pylorus making sure the nasogastric tube is not across the pylorus. The short vessels are then divided and the colon is mobilized away from the pancreas. The proximal jejunum is stapled as well and divided and the root of the mesentery is identified and the vessels are stapled and divided for back bench preparation. The superior mesenteric artery is divided without an aortic patch, at its origin, to avoid injury of the renal arteries and then the pancreas is removed and placed in cold preservation solution on ice.

The kidneys are then retrieved by dividing the aorta, obtaining a large aortic patch cutting the aorta along a line anterior and across the superior mesenteric artery to visualize the posterior internal wall of the aorta for subsequent division of the aortic patch along the lumbar arteries visualizing the renal arterial ostium.

The IVC is divided and the right ureter is identified and slinged as distal as possible to obtain adequate length for the implantation. The patch is fully removed and the right kidney is placed on preservation fluid and ice.

The left kidney is retrieved with the same technique by mobilizing the colon away and obtaining a long ureter for implantation.

In case of small donors, en-bloc retrieval can be considered if the recipient surgical team decides so, and the whole aorta from the SMA to the iliac arteries as well as the IVC from the suprarenal veins to the iliac veins should be retrieved with both ureters with as much length as possible.

The iliac vessels should then be retrieved obtaining as much length as possible in both the internal and external iliac artery and vein avoiding traction at the bifurcation from the common iliac artery to prevent dissection of the intima and perform successful interposition grafts or jump grafts with these vessels.

3.4 TECHNICAL ASPECTS OF RETRIEVAL FROM DCD DONORS

The retrieval procedure in DCD donors is based on the super-rapid technique and involves a rapid laparotomy with aortic cannulation and IVC venting in the abdomen. Once perfusion is undertaken then portal perfusion can be established via direct cannulation of the portal vein, taking care to divide the portal vein to ensure adequate drainage of the pancreas. The remainder is similar to the cold phase dissection in DBD.

3.5 NORMOTHERMIC REGIONAL PERFUSION

Uncontrolled DCD donation has been greatly assisted by the development of normothermic regional perfusion (NRP). NRP is a technique in which instead of removing the abdominal organs rapidly during cold perfusion, a localized abdominal circuit is established through the abdominal aorta and outflow through the IVC; it can also be established through a femoral cannulation. The external circuit is established and oxygenated blood is perfused through the organs whilst in situ. Following the circulation, then in situ cold perfusion is established similar to the non-NRP setting.

By restoring oxygenated blood to the organs, NRP allows organs to recover from anaerobic metabolism and better tolerate subsequent cold storage prior to transplantation. In addition it allows a period of organ assessment using direct visualization and biochemical evaluation of organ function.

3.6 SPECIAL PEDIATRIC CONSIDERATIONS IN MULTIORGAN RETRIEVAL

The ideal donor age range considered for pediatric transplantation is from less than a year to around 50–55 years old, considering all donor characteristics. When considering younger donors, physiological and metabolic immaturity of the donor has to be taken into account as well as higher risk of thrombosis after implantation. In the case of kidney donors, sometimes the kidneys should be retrieved en bloc.

The liver graft should be carefully evaluated at the time of retrieval. As a consideration, steatosis from 30% and higher are routinely used as whole organs, compared to split, where livers should be considered only when steatosis is around or less than 10%.

The split technique in liver transplantation allows the use of left lateral segments from donors to recipients varying between 5 and 30 kg. In recipients less than 5 kg and neonates, further reduction of the left lateral segment may have to be performed. In bigger recipients, segment IV is preserved to increase the liver size utilising the graft as a left lobe (see Figure 3.4).

Splitting a liver can be performed ex situ during bench surgery or in situ during the retrieval operation. In situ has the advantage of reducing the cold ischemia time of both right and left split grafts; however, it requires longer dissection and time at the donor site as well as hemodynamic stability and a more experienced surgical team.

In the case of bowel, the intestine is more susceptible to hypoperfusion either secondary to hypovolemia, hypotension or cardiac arrest in the donor, all leading to ischemic damage, reason why donors with the best hemodynamic parameters

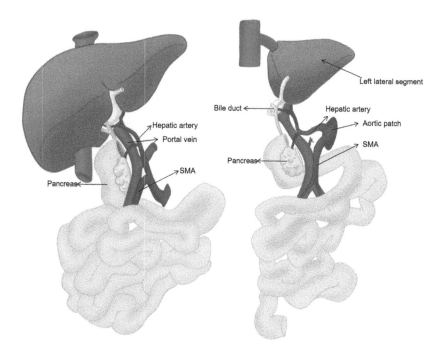

Figure 3.4 The different types of grafts that can be obtained in en-bloc liver pancreas and bowel transplant including reductions of bowel segments in order to optimize size match between donor and recipient.

are best selected as well as in very low inotropic support without any history of heart failure or cardiac arrest.

When transplanting organs in small-weight infants with a background of short gut due to bowel resection and subsequent small cavity, the small-weight donor with a 1–1 ratio can be used. However, a ratio of 1–3 maximum of 1–4 can be reached when the combined graft is reduced. Utilizing the colon in the graft depends in several factors such as size, space in the recipient and anatomical status.

In kidney transplant, the donor selection is also important, like graft function with none to mild dysfunction. Donor and recipient weight ratio is not relevant, only in the case of small donors for big recipients. Using a larger donor on small recipients has the advantage of giving larger parenchymal mass to the recipient. Kidneys from small donors or less than 12–15 kg have a higher risk of thrombosis, these donor kidneys can be used as en bloc in a single large recipient, with the vena cava and aorta of the donor used for anastomosis into the recipient.

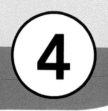

4 Kidney transplantation

Kidney transplantation is the preferred treatment for end-stage renal disease (ESRD) in children; it improves survival, growth, quality of life (QOL) of children and their care holders, as well as neurodevelopment and cognitive function in comparison to dialysis. It has been demonstrated how there is a four times higher risk of death with dialysis than with kidney transplant.

Once the estimated glomerular filtration rate (eGFR) declines, to less than 30 mL/min per 1.73 m², or stage 4 kidney disease, and the child develops chronic kidney disease (CKD), it is time to start preparing both the child and the family for renal replacement therapy (RRT).

4.1 INCIDENCE

In Europe, the estimated median annual incidence of pediatric stage 3 to 5 ESRD is 11.9 cases per million of age-related population (PMARP). In Europe and the United States, congenital causes account for almost 60% of cases of CKD in children. In older children and adolescents, glomerular disease is more prevalent as an underlying cause of CKD.

4.2 ETIOLOGY

In children, the most common causes of ESRD in children are congenital, cystic, and hereditary disease, which account for 35% of incident cases. Glomerulonephritis is the second most common aetiology, accounting for 23% of new cases, predominantly due to focal segmental glomerulosclerosis (FSGS). Secondary glomerulonephritis and vasculitis account for 11% of new cases, of which lupus nephritis is the most common. The underlying aetiology of ESRD also varies by age of presentation. The congenital and structural diseases are more common in the young age groups, while glomerulonephritis is the leading cause in adolescents.

Other causes account for approximately 25% of cases. In 18%, the underlying primary diagnosis may not be identified. Other causes of CKD in children include hemolytic uremic syndrome (HUS), genetic disorders (cystinosis, oxalosis, hereditary nephritis, and Alport syndrome), and interstitial nephritis.

DOI: 10.1201/9781003341741-4

4.3 ADVANTAGES OF KIDNEY TRANSPLANTATION

Patient survival is superior among children with a kidney allograft compared with those who remain on dialysis. Children frequently undergo primary or pre-emptive transplantation, in which transplantation is the first mode of treatment for ESRD. Pre-emptive transplants are performed more frequently in children than adults because of the parents' desire to avoid dialysis when a living donor is available. When performed, this procedure most commonly involves a living donor who is related to the recipient. Children can also be listed for pre-emptive deceased donor transplant.

Previously, ABO incompatibility and the presence of cytotoxic antilympho-cyte antibodies against the donor were contraindications to transplantation; however, subsequent advances with specific protocols have demonstrated successful transplants in some centers.

Kidney paired donation (KPD) or shared scheme, was first conceptualized in the 1980s and provides a method of matching candidates and their willing donors with other candidate-donor pairs such that the resulting transplants are no longer incompatible. This scheme, in pediatrics, is a good alternative in cases where there is ABO mismatch, HLA incompatibility, in the presence of donor-specific antibodies, or even to avoid the risk of exposure to certain viruses.

4.4 TYPES OF DONORS

There is an increasing need for organs in response to an increase number of patients needing a kidney transplant both in the adult population than in the pediatric population. Organ shortage is a global issue. In the UK the majority of pediatric kidney transplants come from Living Donation, either direct donors or by the National Sharing Scheme.

In the UK, the amount of pediatric transplants from living donors is much higher compared than to the US where more transplants come from deceased donors.

The results of kidney transplantation with a living donor are superior to those with a deceased donor. Advantages in transplant timing with living donation increases because dialysis can be avoided, or the period on dialysis can be shortened because the time of transplantation is decided in advance. At the same time, the incidence of delayed allograft function is lower and the long-term survival is higher with living donation.

Living donation has improved the overall outcome of transplant recipients. Timing on is also improved and more pre-dialysis transplants can be performed. At the same time, in the case of complex recipients, or patients with any coexisting iatrogenic or congenital vascular anomalies, living donation should be considered as an alternative.

In the adult population, deceased donation is the most common type of transplantation worldwide; albeit, this is not always seen in children. Whenever the possibility of receiving an organ from the deceased donor pool, several considerations have to be sought in order to accept or decline the offer. There are aspects relevant to the donor history and others related to their background. These donors might well be donors after circulatory death (DCD) or donors after brain death (DBD). The overall shortage of deceased donors for the pediatric population has led to a broad range of efforts to increase donation, including DCD. In the UK deceased donation is very low compared to living donation kidney transplants.

4.5 SURGICAL TECHNIQUE

On admission for transplantation, the patient medical history has to be directed and an extensive physical examination should be performed to ensure there is no immediate contraindication to a major surgery. Immunosuppression is usually commenced early or before the patient goes to surgery. The different type of immunosuppression will be determined depending on the immunological risk factors or the established protocols. In the case viral prophylaxis should be utilized, as well should be given before the surgery.

While the transplant procedure is performed under sterile conditions, the patient will be administered immunosuppressive drugs, which can increase the risk of infections such as wound or urinary tract infections. Additionally, there is a possibility of accidental contamination of the deceased donor kidney during retrieval or the donor having a urinary tract infection due to the presence of a urinary catheter in the intensive care unit. To mitigate these risks, prophylactic antimicrobial therapy is typically provided, targeting common skin organisms and potential urinary tract contaminants.

Although traditionally the right iliac fossa was used for implantation of the kidney, in reality there is little to choose between sides. Implantation should be individualized depending on every patient and also on the size and weight of the recipient. In the case of a small child requiring a kidney transplant into the abdominal cavity, in whom the vascular anastomoses of the renal vessels may be to the aorta and vena cava, the right side of the abdominal cavity is preferred because the kidney is placed behind the cecum and ascending colon.

In recipients whose weight is more than 15–20 kg, there are two common incisions used to expose the external iliac vessels and bladder. The oblique Rutherford Morison or curvilinear incision can be performed, as well as the Alexander or pararectal incision. The external oblique muscle and fascia are divided in the line of the incision and split to the lateral extent of the wound.

The incision is carried to expose the peritoneum and once this is done, the inferior epigastric vessels may be ligated and divided in order to improve access, but if there are multiple renal arteries, these vessels should be preserved in the first instance in case the inferior epigastric artery is required for anastomosis to a lower polar renal artery. The spermatic cord released either side, allowing it to be retracted medially. In females the round ligament can be divided between ligatures.

Depending on whether the transplant renal artery is anastomosed to the common or external iliac artery or whether the carrel patch of the renal artery is anastomosed to either one of the iliac arteries, in the first instance dissection proceeds to expose the external, common, and internal iliac arteries. The lymphatics around the vessels can be preserved where possible and separated from the artery without division. The ones that cross over the artery are carefully ligated and divided to reduce the risk of lymphocele. Having completed the exposure of the appropriate iliac arteries, dissection of the external iliac vein is performed.

In recipients less than 20 kg in weight the right extra peritoneal space can be developed by extending the incision to the right costal margin, or a trans peritoneal approach can be used. The precise weight, at which the preference of incision changes from extra peritoneal to intraperitoneal, varies between different units. In the case of an intraperitoneal approach, the abdomen is opened through a midline incision, and the retro peritoneum opened by incising the peritoneum lateral to the ascending colon which is reflected medially. The terminal portion of the vena cava is dissected over 3–4 cm, ligating and dividing two to three lumbar veins posteriorly. The distal aorta also is dissected free at its bifurcation, as are the proximal ends of the common iliac arteries. Two to three lumbar arteries can be ligated whereas the inferior mesenteric artery (IMA) in protected by passing a sling or a vicryl suture around it twice. A partial occlusion clamp is used to isolate the vena cava first during the venous anastomosis and then the aorta is cross clapped proximally and distally while the blood flow though the IMA is temporarily stopped by pulling gently the previously positioned sling or vicryl suture.

4.6 IMPLANTATION

When the kidney has been prepared and is ready for implantation, the vessels are now ready for clamping. A deceased donor kidney usually has a renal artery or arteries arising from a single aortic patch, and this patch should be trimmed to an appropriate size and used for the anastomosis to the aorta in small children and common iliac artery/external iliac artery for older children. Where there is more than one renal vein, the smaller veins can be ligated, assuming that there is one large renal vein. A short right renal vein can be extended using donor inferior vena cava or iliac vein.

For the arterial anastomosis in patients who are more than 20kg, the donor renal artery is anastomosed to the common or the external iliac arteries end-renal to side-iliac artery with 5–0 or 6–0 monofilament (prolene) vascular suture using the standard anastomotic techniques. For the renal vein, it is anastomosed end-to-side, usually to the external iliac vein using a continuous 5–0 monofilament (prolene) vascular suture, with the initial sutures placed at either end of the venotomy.

When patients are less than 15–20 kg, the renal vein is anastomosed to the vena cava first in an end-to-side technique with non-absorbable monofilament vascular sutures. The renal artery is then anastomosed to the terminal aorta in an end-to-side technique with non-absorbable monofilament vascular sutures.

For the reperfusion, the clamps should be removed in a sequential manner; firstly, the distal clamps in order to allow slow reperfusion of the kidney and identification and correction of significant bleeding before the proximal clamps are released. Careful communication with the anaesthetist is required before removing vascular clamps from the vena cava and aorta, since the perfused kidney requires a large proportion of the patient's circulating volume, resulting in large hemodynamic changes or severe reperfusion injury and the patient needs to be well filled before that.

Once the kidney is reperfused, attention should be paid to controlling significant bleeding points around the anastomoses and ligating any tributaries that were missed while benching the kidney on the back table. It is important to assess the quality of reperfusion after reassuring that all the clamps have been removed, the recipient has a good blood pressure, and there is no intimal dissection of the proximal recipient artery or the donor artery (see Figure 4.1).

Once the kidney has been perfused with recipient blood and hemostasis has been secured, the next step involves reconstructing the urinary tract. The most common method for urinary tract reconstruction is the extra vesical Lich-Gregoir ureteroneocystostomy, which involves connecting the transplant ureter directly to the bladder. The goal is to create an anastomosis between the ureter and the bladder's mucosa, with the distal ureter enclosed in a 2–3 cm tunnel. This design allows for a valve mechanism that prevents urine reflux up to the ureter when the bladder contracts. To reduce the risk of leak and stenosis, a double-pigtail (double-J) ureteric stent is often used, and it is typically removed 4–6 weeks after the transplant.

Another technique employed is the intravesical Politano-Leadbetter approach, where a cystotomy is created to access the interior part of the bladder. The ureter is then introduced into the bladder before closure. In this technique, the urinary catheter remains in place for 4–5 days.

4.7 POSTOPERATIVE CARE

Living donor kidneys will generally function immediately because of the healthy state of the donor as well as the shorter cold ischemic time for the kidney. For deceased donor kidneys, the cold ischemic time is generally longer and there is a higher risk of delayed graft function especially if the kidney is from a donor who died from circulatory death (DCD) instead of brain death (DBD).

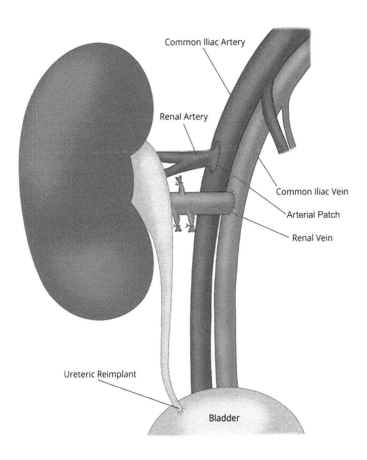

Figure 4.1 Scheme of the kidney transplant implant.

For patients who were oliguric or who had native nephrectomies before transplantation, monitoring urine output is an excellent way of monitoring of graft function in addition to serum creatinine. For patients who made significant urine before transplant, evaluation of graft function can be more difficult. Knowing the baseline urine output before transplant, in addition to the serum creatinine, is the way of monitoring graft function with the expectation that the creatinine should fall during the first 12–24 hours. Recipients with oliguria should be rapidly evaluated. The urinary catheter should be flushed with small volumes of sterile saline. The volume status of the patient should be carefully assessed. A fluid bolus is usually warranted, both as a diagnostic rest and as a therapeutic intervention. Urgent Doppler ultrasonography will confirm adequate arterial flow and venous outflow. Ultrasound will also assess for evidence of fluid or blood around the kidney, as well as the status of the ureter, bladder and ureteric stent for possible ureteral obstruction.

Occasionally there will be a modest reduction in flow suggestive of increased intrarenal resistance, most commonly because of acute tubular necrosis. In instances of renal vein thrombosis, the Doppler will show reverse diastolic flow on the arterial trace and absent flow in the renal vein. The graft will need immediate exploration in this case but it is usually not salvageable. Vascular thrombosis is currently the most common reported cause of early graft loss (EGL), within the first 30 days, and occurs in approximately 5% of kidney transplants.

Although hyperacute or accelerated acute rejections are occasionally responsible for EGL, the most common causes are non-immunological: vascular thrombosis accounts for up to one third of early kidney transplant loss. Primary non-function (PNF) is also important and potential avoidable cause of EGL that may reflect the quality of the donor organ.

Complications related to ureteral anastomosis include leaks and obstruction. The risk of ureteral complications is approximately 7% to 9%. A leak at the ureteral anastomosis generally manifests in the first few days after the transplant. It can present as a collection and a raised creatinine. Obstruction of the urinary system can occur at any time. An early obstruction is usually related to technical problems with the anastomosis or other mechanical issues, such as torsion of the ureter or external compression, while later obstruction often reflects ischemic stricture.

Lymphoceles are other complications after retroperitoneal transplant. They can be asymptomatic, produce discomfort or allograft dysfunction. The diagnosis is established by ultrasound-guided aspiration of clear fluid with a creatinine concentration equivalent to the creatinine in the serum. If elevated, it implies a urine leak.

4.8 OUTCOMES

The type and timing of the transplant affect outcomes. Living donor transplant is associated with a better graft survival compared to deceased donor transplant. Pre-emptive transplantation is associated with better graft survival compared with patients on dialysis at the time of transplantation. For children on dialysis, the choice of dialysis therapy does not impact graft survival compared with patients on dialysis at the time of transplantation. For children on dialysis, the choice of dialysis therapy does not impact graft survival, although graft loss from vascular thrombosis is more common in children on peritoneal dialysis compared with hemodialysis.

Causes of allograft failure following transplantation are chronic rejection (41.3%) vascular thrombosis (8.1%), recurrence of the primary disease (7.9%), acute rejection (6.3%), and discontinuation of immunosuppression (6.3%).

Acute rejection typically occurs between 1 week and 3 months after transplantation, although it can happen at any time. A rise in the serum creatinine level is frequent the first sign of rejection. Any renal dysfunction should be promptly investigated. When other causes have been excluded a percutaneous biopsy should be obtained to confirm the diagnosis. Other causes leading to allograft dysfunction include calcineurin inhibitor toxicity, ureteral obstruction, infection and renal artery stenosis. A biopsy can also diagnose recurrence of the original disease and can be complimented by the use of electron microscopy.

Chronic allograft nephropathy frequently occurs and is the leading cause of graft failure. This process involves both immunological and nonimmunological factors. Although acute rejection episodes are a major risk factor for chronic allograft nephropathy, it is clear other processes can contribute as well. Evidence of antibody-mediated injury is also present in 57% of patients with late allograft dysfunction.

5 Liver transplantation

Pediatric liver transplantation (LT) is an established treatment for end-stage liver disease. However, it is different from adult liver transplantation due to a unique set of challenges. The improved immunosuppression and advanced surgical and anaesthetic techniques have led to expanding the boundaries of the indications. However, the Lack of sized-matched donors poses a major concern in selecting donors. The lack of organs has prompted innovative approaches such as the utilization of split liver grafts, domino transplantation, and increased use of extended criteria donors. Therefore, the decision to use a particular donor organ must strike a balance between the risks associated with the individual liver graft and the risk of the patient's death on the waiting list.

5.1 INDICATIONS FOR LIVER TRANSPLANTATION

Biliary atresia (BA) is the primary indication for pediatric liver transplantation (LT) worldwide. BA is characterized by progressive inflammatory obstruction of both intrahepatic and extrahepatic bile ducts in neonates. While the Kasai portoenterostomy procedure has improved long-term survival, LT remains the ultimate treatment option for patients who have undergone a successful Kasai procedure. Untreated infants with BA face liver cirrhosis, liver failure, or a combination of both within the first year or two of life. Post-Kasai BA patients may require LT due to various indications, such as liver cirrhosis, liver failure, gastrointestinal bleeding, growth retardation, pruritus, intrapulmonary shunting, hepatopulmonary syndrome, and repeated cholangitis.

Alagille syndrome is another cholestatic liver disease affecting the liver and multiple organ systems. Around 20% of children with Alagille syndrome may develop cirrhosis, and a higher percentage experience intractable pruritus. Post-LT outcomes for this group are generally favourable, but attention should be given to potential concomitant heart and intracranial vascular abnormalities.

Progressive familial intrahepatic cholestasis (PFIC) is an autosomal recessive cholestatic disease leading to cirrhosis and necessitating LT. PFIC has three types: PFIC1, PFIC2, and PFIC3. Identifying PFIC is essential after excluding other

DOI: 10.1201/9781003341741-5

major causes of cholestasis. Differentiating PFIC3 is often characterized by high gamma-glutamyl transferase (gamma GT) levels. LT remains crucial for treating PFIC, urea cycle defects, Crigler-Najjar syndrome, homozygous familial hypercholesterolemia, primary hyperoxaluria, and other inborn errors of metabolism that do not injure the liver.

Wilson disease, an autosomal recessive condition, results in acute or chronic liver failure, neurological dysfunction, renal failure, and hemolytic anaemia. Early diagnosis is critical, and LT becomes the elected option when acute or chronic liver failure is present.

Hepatoblastoma is the most prevalent primary liver malignancy in children. With primary resection and chemotherapy, 80% long-term survival rates have been achieved. However, some cases deemed unresectable require LT after neoadjuvant chemotherapy.

The progress made in Hepatoblastoma treatment, combining surgical resection, chemotherapy, and liver transplantation, has significantly improved outcomes and overall quality of life for affected children. Ongoing research and advancements contribute to refining treatment protocols and provide hope for better survival rates in the future.

Acute liver failure requires urgent LT as a lifesaving measure. The low availability of donor livers means that not all patients can receive LT, and the King's College and Clichy-Villejuif criteria help identify patients at the highest risk of death without transplantation. Early detection, timely intervention, and proper treatment planning are vital to enhance survival rates.

5.2 LISTING

During a listing meeting, a multidisciplinary team comprising hepatologists, surgeons, and anaesthetists convenes to evaluate and discuss patients with chronic liver disease who may be suitable candidates for liver transplantation. The primary objective of this meeting is to assess the patients' medical conditions thoroughly, review relevant biochemical data, and determine the necessity of transplantation by comparing the risk of death without a transplant to the risk associated with the procedure.

Critical biochemical data, including serum bilirubin levels, international normalized ratio (INR), and renal function, are pivotal in the decision-making process. To aid in this assessment, predictive equations like the model for end-stage liver disease (MELD) and its UK equivalent, known as UKELD, have been developed. These equations utilize the biochemical data to calculate a numerical score, indicating the severity of the patient's liver disease and their overall risk of mortality.

For instance, a MELD score above 18 or a UKELD score of 49 or higher is considered an indication for liver transplantation. At this stage, the risk of death without transplantation outweighs the risk associated with the procedure. Patients with such scores exhibit a higher survival rate following transplantation compared to the likelihood of survival without the intervention. For example, patients with a UKELD score of 49 have a 9% mortality rate at 1 year if they do not undergo transplantation.

The MELD and UKELD scores are valuable tools for prioritizing patients based on the severity of their liver disease and the urgency of their need for a transplant. Nonetheless, it is essential to recognize that transplantation decisions are intricate and necessitate careful consideration of each patient's unique medical condition and individual circumstances. The Listing meeting serves as a pivotal platform for multidisciplinary collaboration, ensuring that the most suitable candidates are identified and prioritized for liver transplantation, ultimately enhancing the chances of successful outcomes for patients in need.

5.3 TYPES OF DONORS

5.3.1 DECEASED LIVER DONATION

Donors after brain death (DBD) and donors after cardiac death (DCD) are the two primary types of deceased donors. Most liver transplants are performed using grafts from DBD donors. In recent times, the acceptance criteria have broadened considerably, allowing for the utilization of more extended criteria grafts. This includes increased use of DCD grafts (up to 30% in some centers), older and steatotic DBD grafts, grafts with viral challenges, and livers from donors with significant comorbidities. As a result, donor selection and evaluation play a crucial role in ensuring a successful outcome.

When a potential donor is identified, the donor coordinator must meticulously record all pertinent data to determine suitability for donation, with special emphasis on assessing any liver-specific contraindications for donation. The ideal characteristics of DBD liver donors can be described as follows:

1. Age of donor < 50 years

2. Hemodynamically stable

3. Significant inotropic support

4. Sodium < 160 mmol/L

5. AST and ALT < ×5 normal value (possibly higher if falling over previous days)

6. GGT < ×4 normal value

7. BMI < 30

8. ICU stay < 7 or longer if enterally fed

If these criteria are present, the liver should be considered for splitting to match the size of the recipient. Liver splitting for an adult and a pediatric recipient can

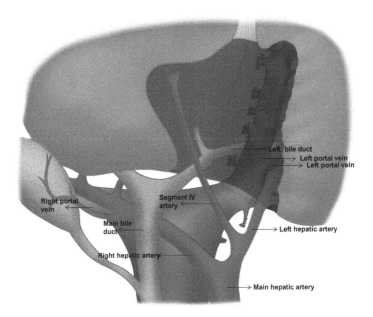

Figure 5.1 Hilar dissection of the left lateral segmentectomy. PV and left hepatic artery are isolated. Note the transection plane (dotted line). PV branches to the seg IV are ligated along the falciform ligament. Lateral branches of the LPV are tied to increase the length of the PV.

also be considered in situations when one of the above criteria is missing, whilst splitting a liver for two adults (full right–full left grafts) should only be considered when all the criteria are met (see Figure 5.1).

Donor after circulatory death grafts

Based on the context in which the cardiac arrest takes place, there are three main categories of organ donors: uncontrolled (Maastricht category I and II), controlled (Maastricht category III), and uncontrolled controlled (Maastricht category IV). These categories differ in several aspects. The controlled group comprises patients in intensive care who have severe and irreversible brain injuries but do not meet the criteria for brainstem death. In this group, life support treatment is withdrawn, leading to cardiac arrest. On the other hand, uncontrolled DCD donors are typically younger individuals with fewer underlying health conditions, and their death occurs due to a sudden and catastrophic cardiac event.

Living donation liver transplant

The shortage of organs has prompted advancements in living donor liver transplantation (LDLT; see Figure 5.2), leading to technical innovations. However,

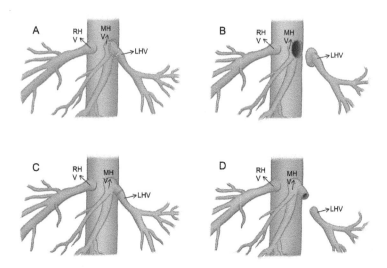

Figure 5.2 Isolation of the LHV in LDLT. In contrast to split liver transplant note the level of transaction of the LHV. In the split liver, transplant opening is much closer to the IVC whereas LDLT it is away from the IVC. Split liver from deceased donor are shown in A and B, living donor left lateral segmentectomy are shown in C and D.

*** RHV – right hepatic vein, MHV – middle hepatic vein, LHV – left hepatic vein.

it is vital to assess potential donors thoroughly to ensure the right patient and graft selection. The mortality risk for living donors is around 0.1–0.3%, with a complication risk of 15–20%. Hence, LDLT should only be performed when the potential benefits to the recipient outweigh the risks to the donor. A high BMI (> 30) is not an absolute barrier for living donation. Evidence suggests that intensive diet and exercise programs can help donors reach the desired BMI target and reduce liver steatosis. Conversely, some centers have successfully implemented weight gain programs for donors to ensure an adequate liver mass for the recipient and reduce the risk of small-for-size syndrome.

Donor surgery for liver transplantation is a critical procedure that requires an experienced surgeon with a profound understanding of liver anatomy. Pre-operative imaging is crucial to identify any anatomical variations that may affect decision-making during the surgery. The procedure can be performed using an open, laparoscopic, or robotic approach, with a growing trend towards robotic donor hepatectomy.

During the surgery, the left lateral segment of the liver is mobilized, and the left hepatic vein is carefully released. An intraoperative cholangiogram is often performed to visualize the bile duct anatomy. The dissection of the hilum follows, with attention given to the artery and portal vein supplying the left lateral segment. Parenchymal transection is then carried out to remove the left lateral segment, and the level of transection is determined based on the division of the bile duct.

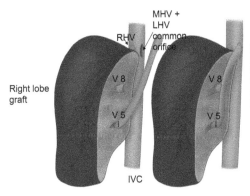

Figure 5.3 Segment V and VIII reconstructions in LDLT. In cases with a donation of the left lobe with the middle hepatic vein, donor segment V and VIII keep undrained and may lead to congestion, in order to prevent congestion and graft failure. reconstruction of the seg V and VIII is being done. The picture demonstrates the reconstruction of Seg V and VIII using vein graft to make A SINGLE outflow in the IVC while seg VIII is connected at the middle. Instead, if the Seg VIII is very close to the IVC it can make a common opening with seg V graft.

*** IVC – Inferior vena cava, RHV – right hepatic vein, LHV – left hepatic vein, RHV – right hepatic vein, V5 – segment 5 vein, V8 – segment 8 vein.

Preserving the right duct is essential to ensure successful transplantation outcomes and preserve optimal liver function for both the donor and recipient. Donor surgery demands precision, expertise, and a comprehensive understanding of liver anatomy. The safety and well-being of the donor are paramount, and careful planning and execution are critical to achieving successful liver transplantation outcomes for both parties involved.

In a full left lobe donation for liver transplantation, the dissection process is similar to that of the left lateral segment (LLS) donation, but with some additional considerations. One debated aspect in this procedure is whether to include the middle hepatic vein (MHV) with the graft or not.

If the decision is made to include the MHV with the graft, it becomes essential to reconstruct the branches of segments V and VIII in the liver remnant left in the donor's body (Figure 5.3). This reconstruction is necessary to ensure the safety and functionality of the remaining liver tissue. By reconstructing these branches, the blood supply to the remnant liver is optimized, reducing the risk of complications and promoting better liver regeneration and function in the donor.

The choice of including the MHV or not in the graft depends on various factors, including the anatomical characteristics of the donor's liver, the recipient's condition, and the surgical team's expertise. Each case must be carefully assessed,

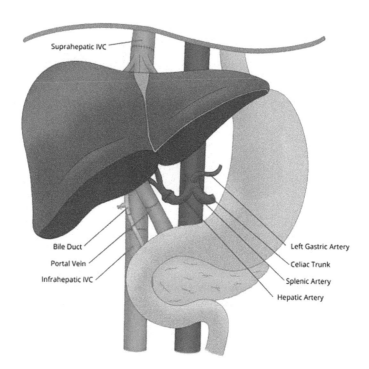

Figure 5.4 Liver transplantation with whole liver graft with caval replacement.

and the decision should be made in the best interest of both the donor and the recipient (see Figure 5.4).

The ultimate goal of full left lobe donation is to provide a healthy and sufficient graft for the recipient while ensuring the donor's safety and well-being. The surgical team must thoroughly evaluate the vascular anatomy of the donor liver and plan the dissection and reconstruction meticulously to achieve successful outcomes for both parties involved in the transplantation process.

5.3.1.1 Types of grafts

There are various types of grafts used in pediatric liver transplantation, and choosing the right graft size is essential to avoid complications like small-for-size syndrome (SFSS). The main types of grafts used are as follows:

1. *Whole liver graft*: This involves transplanting the entire liver from a deceased donor into the recipient. It is commonly used in older and larger pediatric patients who need a larger liver volume to support their metabolic needs.

2. *Split liver graft*: The liver from a deceased donor is divided into two segments, which can be transplanted into two recipients. This allows one donor liver to be

used for both an adult and a pediatric patient or two pediatric patients, expanding the donor pool and increasing transplant opportunities.

3. *Living donor graft*: In this procedure, a healthy living donor, usually a close family member, donates a portion of their liver, which is then transplanted into the pediatric recipient. Both the donor and recipient liver segments grow back to their original size after surgery.

To avoid SFSS, which occurs when the graft size is inadequate for the recipient's metabolic demands, selecting the appropriate graft size is crucial. Smaller grafts should typically be at least 40% of the standard liver volume or have a graft-to-recipient weight ratio (GRWR) of 0.8. GRWR is an important parameter used to assess the suitability of the graft size relative to the recipient's body weight. It ensures the safety and success of pediatric liver transplantation with smaller grafts.

Choosing the correct graft size is critical in pediatric liver transplantation to achieve optimal outcomes, minimize complications, and promote long-term graft survival and recipient well-being. The decision on the graft type and size is based on a thorough evaluation of the recipient's medical condition, age, size, and the availability of suitable donors. Close collaboration among the transplant team and a comprehensive assessment are crucial factors in achieving successful outcomes in pediatric liver transplantation.

5.3.1.1.1 Split liver transplant

This procedure allows transplanting two patients with a single cadaveric organ, usually a child and adult. The partition is usually performed ex situ, producing a left lateral segment graft for a small recipient (pediatric) and an extended right graft for an adult (Figure 5.5). More recently, attempts were made to transplant two adults creating a right and a left lobe graft, although the results are not as good as for the child and adult split.

5.3.1.2 Recipient procedure

The transplant procedure is divided into three phases; hepatectomy, the anhepatic phase and, implantation. The hepatectomy is a difficult technical procedure and the approach needs to be flexible. It requires an experienced surgeon, familiar with different types of liver grafts: split, LDLT, or a potential domino LT. The hepatectomy with inferior vena cava excision is an approach in which the IVC is excised with the native liver, controlling the supra and infra-hepatic ends of the IVC. This interrupts the venous return with subsequent reduction in the cardiac output, congestion of all abdominal organs and lower limbs, and significant hemodynamic changes. An alternative is to use the veno-venous bypass, shunting the intrahepatic IVC as well as the portal vein in the axillary or internal jugular veins. Though more physiological, this technique is associated with air embolism,

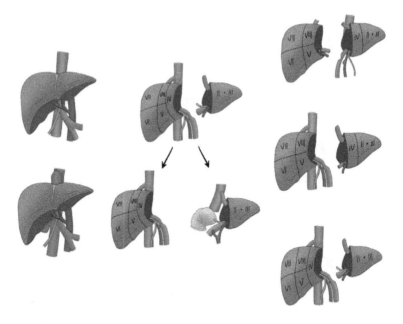

Figure 5.5 Couinaud segments of the left lateral segment and left lobe grafts. LLS includes segments II and III, while the left lobe includes II, III, and IV with or without MHV. Right lobe graft includes V, VI, VII, VIII +/–IV.

coagulopathy, risk of pleural puncture, and axillary and or groin seroma/infection, especially in the adult population.

The piggyback technique, hepatectomy with IVC preservation, is a technique that allows preservation of the retro hepatic IVC by means of complete mobilization of the liver until only the hepatic veins remain connected. To achieve this, it is particularly helpful to disconnect the hepatic hilum, which effectively means interrupting the portal venous flow. A temporary portocaval shunt should be created in these cases to enable hemodynamic stability, avoid small bowel congestion and allow the assessment of the portal flow.

5.3.1.3 Implantation

Caval replacement transplant. The suprahepatic caval anastomosis is undertaken first followed by the infrahepatic one, avoiding leaving an excessive length of donor cava. At this point, the graft can be flushed through the portal vein with a ringer or saline to avoid hyperkalaemia after reperfusion. If veno-venous bypass is used, this is disconnected at this stage. An end-to-end portal-venous (PV) anastomosis is then performed, by deliberately performing the knot away from the vessel, hence leaving a growth factor for the vein to distend once flow is re-established to avoid stenosis.

Piggyback implantation. This can be undertaken as a side-to-side anastomosis between the donor and recipient IVC or anastomosing the suprahepatic end of the donor IVC to the hepatic veins. The graft can be flushed through the portal vein. In both cases, the infra-hepatic end of the donor IVC will be closed.

Arterial anastomosis is then performed. Depending on the graft, a suitable area of anastomosis is determined after matching the diameter of the donor artery and recipient hepatic artery (HA). Sometimes it may require multiple anastomoses. Then the bile duct anastomosis is performed as hepaticojejunostomy or duct-to-duct.

5.3.1.4 Portal hypertension, shunt ligation, and ligation of splenic artery in pediatric liver transplantation

Portal hypertension is a condition that arises from the distortion of liver architecture caused by cirrhosis. This distortion obstructs the normal flow of portal venous blood, leading to an increase in pressure within the portal circulation. As portal hypertension progresses, the body compensates by developing new collateral channels that divert blood from the portal system to the systemic venous system. These collaterals can form along the peritoneal attachments of the liver, such as the ligament teres, and may present as varices around the gastro-oesophageal junction.

During liver transplantation, these collateral vessels and the abnormal clotting cascade associated with portal hypertension account for a significant portion of bleeding complications. Manifestations of portal hypertension include gastrointestinal bleeding, ascites (accumulation of fluid in the abdominal cavity), hypersplenism (overactive spleen), and encephalopathy (brain dysfunction). To address portal hypertension, the focus of treatment is on preventing complications.

Porto pulmonary hypertension is another consequence of portal hypertension, characterized by an elevated resting mean pulmonary artery pressure (greater than 25 mm Hg). In severe cases, with mean pulmonary artery pressure exceeding 50 mm Hg, the cardiopulmonary mortality rate approaches 100%. During liver transplantation, evaluating portal vein (PV) flow is crucial, and some centers perform real-time measurements of PV flow and pressure to avoid inaccuracies and miscalculations.

To improve portal flow and prevent subclinical encephalopathy after liver transplantation, it is essential to ligate the shunts created by the collateral vessels. Additionally, ligation of the splenic artery may be necessary in cases where the cirrhotic liver's PV flow poses a risk to the new liver graft, especially if the graft is marginal in size. By addressing these issues related to portal hypertension during liver transplantation, the chances of successful outcomes and graft survival can be significantly improved.

5.3.1.5 Domino liver transplant

The domino liver transplantation is an innovative surgical technique that utilizes a graft from a recipient with a metabolic liver-based defect, like Familial Amyloid Polyneuropathy (FAP), but with otherwise normal liver function. This approach addresses the organ shortage and benefits multiple patients in need of liver transplantation.

In this procedure, the liver from a donor with the metabolic defect is transplanted into a "domino recipient." The graft comes from an individual with relatively unaffected liver function, making it suitable for transplantation. The "domino recipient" receives this graft, potentially improving or stabilizing their metabolic condition while maintaining good liver function.

Subsequently, the recipient's explanted liver, affected by the metabolic disorder, can be transplanted into another patient, known as the "second recipient." This is particularly advantageous for patients with advanced liver disease or cancer, as the risk of metabolic disorder manifestations in the "second recipient" is relatively low compared to waiting for a conventional liver graft.

The domino liver transplantation offers both the "domino recipient" and the "second recipient" the opportunity for a functional liver, addressing the organ shortage and optimizing transplant opportunities for patients with specific metabolic liver-based defects.

The procedure can be performed using either the classic technique or a piggyback approach. The classic technique involves removing the recipient's diseased liver and transplanting the domino liver in the standard anatomical position. The piggyback approach retains the recipient's native liver while placing the domino liver above it, suitable for certain cases.

Overall, the domino liver transplantation represents a significant advancement in liver transplantation, expanding the use of viable donor livers and improving the prognosis for patients with metabolic disorders. This innovative strategy holds promise in meeting the organ shortage challenge and improving transplant outcomes for those in need.

5.3.1.6 Complications

Liver transplantation is a lifesaving procedure, but it is not without risks. Within the first year after transplantation, there is a 5–10% mortality rate, with most deaths occurring during the early postoperative care period. Therefore, meticulous monitoring, a multidisciplinary approach, and a thorough understanding of the chronological events are crucial for ensuring the best possible outcomes.

Continuous monitoring of the liver post-transplant is essential to detect any signs of deterioration that may indicate complications. Biochemical monitoring using serum markers of liver function is an important tool in assessing the health of the transplanted liver.

Surgical complications following liver transplantation can be nonspecific, such as bleeding, wound infection, wound breakdown, atelectasis, pneumonia, and pleural effusion. Additionally, biliary complications are relatively common, occurring in approximately 10–20% of liver transplant recipients. These complications may manifest as bile leakage or an anastomotic stricture, with the majority presenting within the first 3 months after transplantation. Late complications, mainly strictures, are less common.

Notably, split liver transplants tend to have a higher incidence of early complications compared to whole liver transplants. Several risk factors contribute to the development of biliary complications. These factors include the quality of the arterial blood supply, ABO incompatibility between the donor and recipient, prolonged cold ischemia time (time during which the organ is without blood flow), biliary tree infections, recurrence of the underlying liver disease, and the use of donors after circulatory death (DCD donors).

To minimize the risk of complications and improve patient outcomes, liver transplant teams must remain vigilant in their postoperative care, promptly identify any issues that arise, and promptly initiate appropriate interventions.

One of the arterial complications that may occur early post-transplant is hepatic artery thrombosis (HAT). HAT usually manifests with a sudden clinical deterioration and concomitant worsening of liver biochemistry. In the pediatric setting, hepatic artery thrombosis can occur in up to 30% of cases. The consequences of HAT depend on the time of presentation. Thrombosis in the late postoperative period, months or years after transplant, may present more insidiously with biliary complications or liver abscess formation. In contrast, hepatic artery stenosis may also present with biliary complications in the early post-transplant period.

Venous outflow problems are usually secondary to a suprahepatic vena caval anastomotic stenosis when a classical caval replacement technique has been used for transplant. Presentation is with marked ascites and lower limb oedema. Diagnosis is by measuring a pressure gradient across the anastomosis, and balloon angioplasty is the treatment of choice.

Portal vein thrombosis (PVT) is unusual but may occur early post-transplant, particularly in patients with a prior portal or mesenteric venous thrombosis. PVT is less common than HAT and is almost always a technical complication (1–2%). The portal vein should be optimized by ligating the previous portosystemic shunts (spontaneous or surgical) to improve portal flow. Late PVT will produce signs of portal hypertension with almost no effect on graft function. However, acute thrombosis can cause graft failure with raised enzymes.

Pseudoaneurysms occur late after liver transplantation in approximately 2% of patients. The most common location is at the level of the donor-recipient arterial anastomosis, while a less common site is at the site of ligation of the donor gastroduodenal artery. Pseudoaneurysms can be caused by infection or technical failure and should be treated promptly to prevent heavy bleeding.

Medical complications of liver transplantation can be early or late. All the well-recognized general medical complications seen after major surgery, including cardiac decompensation, electrolyte disturbances, and renal dysfunction, can also occur post-transplant. Additionally, acute rejection is common in the early post-transplant period but rarely causes long-term damage. Rejection is usually cell-mediated, although antibody-mediated rejection may also occur.

5.3.1.7 Theatre setup

We have experience in adult and pediatric liver transplants since the 1990s, and this includes pediatric living donor-related, small bowel, and multivisceral transplants. There is a designated theatre with a multidisciplinary team of surgeons, anaesthetists, clinical perfusion scientists, recipient transplant co-ordinators, registered nurses, operating department practitioners, and healthcare assistants. They rotate in hepatobiliary surgery, multiorgan retrievals, and transplantations to foster experience in all aspects of liver surgery. This promotes a standard of care to the patients by the team and training for all staff. a senior operating department assistant (SODP), two registered and a senior healthcare assistants will staff the theatre at all times.

Teamwork is important to promote cohesion at work and to maintain high-level skills and competencies. The unit would be audited by the CQC, HTA and the National Health Service Blood and Transfusion (NHSBT) for NOR. All theatre staff must be trained to scrub for multi organ retrievals and as an operating perfusion practitioner (OPP). Staff development programmes and courses can help with career progression, recruitment, and retention.

The theatre must be spacious enough to accommodate all theatre equipment as well as specialist equipment like an argon diathermy unit, suction, a cavitron ultrasonic surgical aspirator (CUSA), an intraoperative ultrasound, a warming mattress, a cell saver, and a rapid infuser (see Figure 5.6). Instrument sets for transplants and hepatobiliary surgery include microvascular instruments and

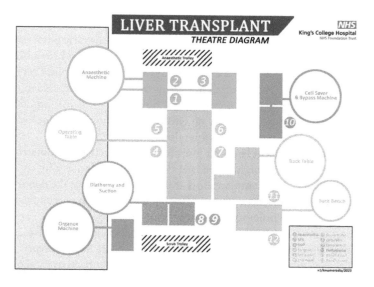

Figure 5.6 Liver transplant theatre diagram.

Thompson retractors, which are used at all times for all transplants and other surgical procedures.

All consumables from swabs to hemostatic sealants should be available at all times in the theatre. At the end of the day/shift, the theatre is prepped and set up for emergencies and transplants at all times.

There must be an HTA accredited refrigerator to store cadaveric iliac vessels, superior mesenteric veins, and aorta. Cadaveric fascia for abdominal wall transplant to facilitate closure, are also stored in the same fridge. The refrigerator's temperature is controlled between 2 and 8 degrees Celslus and is checked daily by the theatre staff as well as remotely monitored 24/7.

It is important to maintain the well-being and mental health of all personnel by being aware of when staff is struggling and giving them access to help from professional bodies, such as occupational health and counselling services. Arranging get togethers either at work or outside can promote teamwork.

5.3.1.8 Anaesthetics

As has been detailed, there is surgical nuance and complexity for surgical mechanics with this cohort of pediatric patients. What must also be at the forefront of any transplantation team is the perioperative preparedness and intraoperative expertise of the physicians and allied healthcare staff. Liver transplantation in particular is not simply an extended practice for pediatric anaesthetists. Nursing and perfusion staff cannot simply be borrowed from other areas. If a service is to run to low morbidity/mortality outcomes, then, much like surgeons, they need to be bespoke.

5.3.1.8.1 Bespoke teams

In order to be a world leader transplant unit, deep understanding of all the areas of transplantation is a cornerstone, in order to optimise outcomes. To enable mastery, a small number of specialist anaesthetists carry out all adult, pediatric, and neonatal transplants, covering 24-hour periods with the help of single speciality ODPs/ Anaesthesia nurses with bespoke trained perfusion scientists. There needs to be this saturation in the case type to enable excellence of nuanced techniques and clear understanding of operative options by phase to enable correct decision-making.

5.3.1.8.2 Location

Specific theatres dedicated to transplantation allow ergonomic placement of equipment, reducing error and improving technical skills. A familiar patient pathway is developed, hardwiring a part of the patient journey, and broadening the cerebral bandwidth of clinicians to allow better clinical performance.

5.3.2 PREASSESSMENT

Accurate, well-considered patient selection remains the cornerstone of successful transplantation. The collaboration of hepatologists, surgeons, anaesthetists, and pediatricians is crucial in making decisions. A well-attended, time-protected, job-planned meeting allows decisions on:

- Preoperative optimization (physiology/pharmacology)
- Need for collaborative institution working (cardiac center involvement)
- Need for additional equipment (ventilators/vascular access)
- Need for additional blood products (coagulopathies/antibodies)
- Optimal timing (daytime hours)

5.3.3 VASCULAR ACCESS

A primary transplant in an otherwise physically well, greater than 10 Kg child is a different proposition to a sub-2Kg, fulminant, coagulopathy, syndromic neonate. As such, one package of vascular access clearly doesn't fit all.

There are, however, common lessons. A degree of calm pragmatism is needed. What you want in terms of venous and arterial access is sometimes (often) not what you can attain. A wide range of devices and techniques of insertion are needed. A flexibility in insertion site, subclavian/jugular/femoral for central venous, is useful to aid success.

Most people advocate in plane (or out of plane) dynamic use of ultrasound to assist vessel location and line passage.

There is a variety of ultrasound machines and probes, but we find the pediatric "hockey stick" to be a peerless allrounder.

In terms of number and size of venous lines, there is no standard recipe. Certainly a multi-lumen central venous line should be seen as mandatory to guide fluid replacement and enable safe use of oft-needed vasoactive infusions. It is commonplace to have to line up multiple infusions on a single available lumen; downstream placement of noradrenaline is recommended if this is the case.

Arterial access is slightly more controversial. It is of course ideal to have continued invasive monitoring of an often-labile blood pressure (over a non-invasive DINAMAP) although there are occasions when it is technically impossible. The decision to continue or not with a transplant under these circumstances should rest with the operative team.

As small a device as possible is preferable to avoid distal flow insufficiency, and avoiding an end artery without alternate supply is widely agreed to be good practice. Other than that, it comes down to anesthesia preference.

5.3.4 INTRAOPERATIVE MONITORING

In recent years, the prevalence in the use of the EEG (electroencephalogram) and NIRS (near-infrared spectroscopy) has increased, in some centers so much so as to become a standard of care. The EEG is certainly useful when using TIVA regimes (especially in the fulminant pediatric cohort where avoidance of volatile agents seems cerebrally protective through lack of vascular-CO_2 decoupling) are used. NIRS can be an excellent non-invasive tool to more rapidly identify reduced oxygen delivery through occult/underappreciated blood loss.

5.3.5 INTRAOPERATIVE MANAGEMENT OF BLOOD LOSS

Blood loss can be both predictably and unpredictably torrential (>250 mL/kg^{-1}). The key to successful resuscitation is a combination of anticipation (availability of products/sufficient calibre vascular access/appropriate additional manpower) and activity.

It is of course obvious that smaller children have smaller intravascular volumes; it is however not always easy to appreciate the developed implication of smaller visual blood loss – a combination of swabs, collections in surgical drapes, and non-cell salvage suction can mean easily losing track of significant blood loss in these cases.

Best attempts at monitoring losses through diligent process of weighing swabs (tare weights), single collection suction, and clear communication is paramount. We suggest having a dedicated individual (a perfusion scientist, ideally) to focus on cell salvage (ACD/heparin preservate) along with a pre-alerted highly co-operative hematology/transfusion service.

We use packed red cells to replace red cell loss, although there may be movement to whole blood in future years if various trials (mainly military and pre-hospital) show benefits without risks/side effects. It is important to remember that using PRC and cell salvage blood will quickly become depleted. Attempt to use empirical or point-of-care-guided major hemorrhage protocols wherever possible. We find TEG to be especially useful, and we find using a system that extrapolates data to estimate fibrinogen levels to be especially useful.

For massive and hyper massive hemorrhage, specific factor concentrates may be needed to regain coagulation control. We advise liaisoning with coagulation hematologists before use of factor VII, Beriplex, or other synthetic factor concentrates.

There is some debate about the importance and timing (pre-/post-implantation) of platelet transfusion in the maintenance of coagulation hemostasis. That said, maintaining both primary and secondary functional coagulation integrity is crucial for both graft survival and reduction in quantity of blood loss.

Remember that hepatic artery thrombosis is a major cause of graft dysfunction. Although polyfactorial, overtransfusion of PRCs to hyperviscosity or unnecessary transfusion of coag factors will certainly contribute to the incidence. Target-guided transfusion will go some way to helping avoid morbidity.

5.3.6 DRUG INFUSIONS

There are many well published guidelines about critical care infusions. We run Noradrenaline infusions early, as there is some evidence that it reduces splanchnic blood loss during transplantation. A fixed concentration protocol by body weight reduces error in rate calculation, but means care should be taken with heavier children who will occasionally have very "strong" vasoactive syringe mixes (0.3 uk/kg^{-1} body weight/50 mL diluent = 0.1 ug/kg/min^{-1} *per mL/hr^{-1} infusion*).

5.3.7 ROLE OF THE ANESTHETIC NURSING STAFF

To have successful results for pediatric liver, small bowel, and multivisceral transplants, there needs to be a standardized process in place with highly experienced and skilled anaesthetic practitioners. There needs to be in-depth knowledge of the stages of a transplant to ascertain what may be required to keep the patient stable. There needs to be good, open, and constant communication between all team members.

Firstly, the patient is anaesthetized via their cannula. For the patient's airway the standard is for ETT microcuff, fixated with elastoplast trousers and the patient also requires NG tube insertion. Eyes are secured with a Jelonet dressing to protect them. An arterial line is then placed, usually radial. A central line is inserted, normally in the right internal jugular vein. The central line needs to have multiple lumens and of large gauges so as to be able to give vasopressors and high volumes of fluid. If a complex pediatric with high blood loss expected then a percutaneous sheath will also be inserted.

The fluid set up is X1 Gelofusine 500 mL bag ran through a hotline and X1 NACL 250 mL also run through a hotline, both connected with three-way taps and an extension to go to the main fluid line. Both using blood giving sets and labeled with a yellow sticker on the Gelofusine line and a red sticker on the NACL line. This is to allow the anaesthetist to bolus 50 mL of their chosen fluid at a time.

The patient then needs to be positioned and pressures areas well protected, as the cases are likely to be a minimum of 8 hours. This is done by wrapping softban wool and crepe around the heels and knees. The arms are protected using softban and incopads. The patient remains normothermic by using a Bair Hugger and blankets. The head is protected with a horseshoe/head ring and insulated with an incopad wrapped around.

A baseline blood gas, TEG, full blood count, and clotting is required. This is to see if anything needs to be corrected at the very beginning of the transplant. These need to be repeated at dissection, anhepatic, and reperfusion stages. Often, blood gas and TEG are more frequent and done hourly, depending on the complexity of the surgery.

It is important to ensure blood products are available at the beginning of the transplant, should they be needed; the standard ordering for a pediatric under 10 kg is ×2 adult packed red cells, ×2 Octaplas and ×1 platelets. For above 10 kg the standard ordering is ×4 adult packed red cells, ×4 Octaplas and ×1 platelets.

For anesthetic practitioners it is important to be more alert at the dissection phase, as the patient could require more blood products if there is bleeding due to previous surgery, since most pediatric cases are due to biliary atresia and so have had a Kasai procedure previously. The patient needs to be well filled to perfuse the donor liver upon reperfusion. Reperfusion phase is the most critical stage of a transplant for anaesthetic practitioners, as the patient could arrest at this point. Therefore, the team will need to be on high alert to support the anaesthetist for an optimal outcome. Indeed, excellent teamwork with good levels of communication and highly competent individuals is the key to success.

6 Pancreas transplantation

Type 1 diabetes mellitus (DM1) is an autoimmune disease in which the pancreatic islet insulin-producing beta cells are selectively destroyed. It most commonly presents in childhood and continues to represent a therapeutic challenge. Secondary diabetes complications, observed in 30% to 50% of patients who live more than 20 years after onset of the disease, result in poor QOL, premature death, and high healthcare costs. The principal determinant of the risk of devastating diabetes complication is the total lifetime exposure to elevated blood glucose levels.

Pancreas transplantation in the pediatric age group is uncommon, and most are in diabetic children who also have renal failure and thus need kidney transplantation, obligating them to immunosuppression. In this group, the outcomes are such that it seems reasonable to recommend the addition of the pancreas so that the child can become insulin independent as well as dialysis free. For non-uremic diabetic children with extreme liability to hypoglycaemic events, in whom successful pancreas transplantation would be appropriate treatment, the antirejection strategies need to be optimized to improve the graft survival rates versus what has been achieved in the past. With respect to outcome measures other than insulin independence, prevention and reversal of secondary complications, improvement in quality of life, extension of life span, and reduction of healthcare costs per quality-adjusted life-year have all been positively demonstrated in type 1 diabetic pancreas recipients. In patients with labile diabetes and hypoglycaemic unawareness, pancreas transplantation can resolve an otherwise intractable and life-threatening course. A variety of surgical techniques have been used for pancreas transplantation and in particular the management of the exocrine secretions and venous drainage of pancreas.

There are three categories of pancreas transplantation recipients:

1. Uremic diabetic patients who undergo a simultaneous pancreas and kidney transplantation from a deceased donor or rarely forma living donor.

2. Nephropathic patients who already have had renal insufficiency corrected, usually by living donor kidney transplantation, and then undergo a pancreas after kidney (PAK) transplantation.

3. Non-uremic diabetic patients who undergo a pancreas transplantation alone (PTA).

DOI: 10.1201/9781003341741-6

6.1 DONOR OPERATION

The majority of pancreas grafts are procured from multiorgan deceased donors, and because the liver and pancreas share the origins of their arterial blood supply, a whole organ pancreas graft usually requires reconstruction. The blood supply to the tail of the pancreas is supplied by the splenic artery, originating from the celiac axis, and the head of the pancreas is supplied by the pancreaticoduodenal arcades, originating from the superior mesenteric artery and the hepatic artery. The usual approach is to use an arterial Y-graft of the donor iliac vessels as a conduit. This is done by anastomosing the internal iliac artery to the graft splenic artery and the external iliac artery to the graft superior mesenteric artery, leaving the common iliac artery segment of the Y-graft to anastomose to the recipient arterial system, usually the right common iliac artery. The portal vein of the donor is usually divided midway between the upper border of the pancreas and the liver, leaving adequate length for transplantation of both organs. If necessary, an extension graft of donor iliac vein can be anastomosed to the pancreatic graft portal vein portion to elongate this.

6.2 IMPLANTATION

In the recipient, the pancreas graft's portal vein, with or without an extension graft, can be connected to either the systemic venous system (usually the iliac vein or vena cava) or to the portal system (usually the superior mesenteric vein). Generally, connecting to the recipient iliac vein is the preferred method. When the venous drainage is directed to the recipient iliac vein, the whole pancreas graft can be oriented with the head directed either into the pelvis or the upper abdomen. If directed cephalically, enteric drainage is the only option. When directed caudally, the duodenum can be anastomosed to the bladder or bowel.

In the bladder-drainage technique, the anastomosis can be hand-sewn or less commonly performed with an end-to-end anastomosis stapler (EEA) brought through the distal duodenum for connection to the post of the anvil projected through the posterior bladder by an anterior cystostomy. The inner layer is then reinforced with a running absorbable suture for hemostasis and to bury the staples under the mucosa. With enteric drainage, which is the most common method, the bowel anastomosis may be hand-sewn in a two-layer end-to-side fashion, or it can be done in a side-to-side fashion by hand-sewing or using an EEA stapler inserted into the end of the graft duodenum, with the post projected through the side wall. The anvil is inserted into the recipient bowel through an enterotomy secured around the connecting post by a purse-string suture. The two posts are connected, and the stapler is fired to create the anastomosis. The end of the duodenum is then closed with a simple stapler. The hand-sewn technique is again the most common method used.

The enteric anastomosis can be directly anastomosed to the most convenient proximal small bowel loop of the recipient or to a Roux-en-Y segment of the

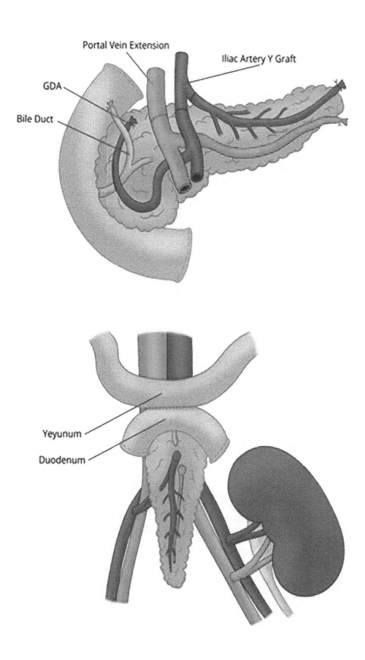

Figure 6.1 Pancreatic transplant and kidney transplant on the same recipient.

recipient's bowel that is created at the time. Outcome analyses do not show any statistical advantage of a Roux-en-Y loop. The choice of technique may depend on the surgeon's preference and the specific clinical situation (see Figure 6.1).

6.3 OUTCOMES

A study of 30,000 pancreatic transplants in the United States has provided valuable insights into patient and graft survival rates following primary pancreas transplantation in the adult population. At the one-year mark, survival rates were reported to be 96% for simultaneous pancreas-kidney (SPK) recipients, 97% for pancreas after kidney (PAK) recipients, and 97% for pancreas transplant alone (PTA) recipients. These rates slightly decreased at the three-year mark to 92%, 91%, and 92%, respectively. Notably, PTA recipients exhibited the highest patient survival rate, suggesting that this group may have had fewer complications before transplantation.

Examining the primary pancreas graft survival rates at one year, the study found rates of 85% for SPK recipients, 79% for PAK recipients, and 78% for PTA recipients. By the three-year mark, the graft survival rates decreased to 79%, 68%, and 62%, respectively. Among the recipient categories, the SPK group showed the highest pancreas graft survival rates, likely attributed to the presence of a kidney graft, enabling earlier detection of rejection episodes compared to the other categories where only the pancreas can be monitored.

Detection of pancreas allograft rejection episodes involves specific criteria. In enteric-drained grafts, rejection may be indicated by a transient rise in serum amylase or lipase, while in bladder-drained grafts, a decline in urine amylase may be suggestive of rejection. In SPK transplantation, a rise in serum creatinine could be an indicator of rejection. To confirm these episodes, a biopsy of the pancreas graft can be performed.

The study also shed light on surgical complications associated with pancreas transplantation. The most frequent complication leading to graft loss was venous or arterial thrombosis, occurring in 5% to 10% of cases. Reoperation was also relatively common, reported in 30% of cases. Anastomotic leaks could occur and be associated with rejection in some instances. Early diagnosis may allow graft salvage, but graft excision is often the preferred treatment to expedite recovery.

In this series, the majority of recipients were over 15 years old, while only three patients were under 15 years old. However, it is noteworthy that a significant percentage of organs used for SPK (7%) and PAK (6%) and 15% for PTA came from donors under 15 years old.

Overall, these findings underscore the significance of meticulous monitoring and early detection of complications after pancreas transplantation. Regular evaluation of graft function and patient well-being is crucial to ensure the best possible outcomes for pancreas transplant recipients.

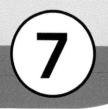

7

Islet cell transplantation

Islet cell transplantation is a rare procedure in children and is typically performed as a follow-up to total pancreatectomy with islet cell auto transplantation. However, this procedure comes with its own set of complications, both in the short and long term.

Islet cell transplantation is a well-established approach for treating diabetes resulting from pancreatectomy performed for chronic pancreatitis or for type 1 diabetes with severe hypoglycaemia and glycaemic instability. Chronic pancreatitis can significantly impair a patient's quality of life, leading to debilitating pain, frequent hospitalizations, and an increased risk of opioid dependence. Total pancreatectomy is selectively indicated in certain cases, and islet transplantation is aimed at enhancing the patient's quality of life and restoring insulin function.

In the management of children with chronic pancreatitis, various surgical techniques have been described to alleviate pain and improve their quality of life. These approaches may involve specific resections or drainage procedures with various variations. While pain relief is achieved in around 50% of patients, many of them still develop endocrine and exocrine insufficiency over time. Therefore, finding the most effective and suitable surgical management for these young patients remains a challenge.

Overall, islet cell transplantation in children is a valuable strategy in select cases of chronic pancreatitis and type 1 diabetes, but it is not without risks and complications. The procedure is intended to improve the patient's overall well-being, reduce pain, and restore insulin function. However, careful consideration and ongoing research are essential to optimize outcomes and minimize long-term complications for these young patients.

7.1 SURGICAL TECHNIQUE FOR AUTO TRANSPLANTATION

The primary distinction between islet auto transplantation in adults and children lies in the focus on minimizing warm ischemia time and maximizing the preservation of islet cells. This objective is achieved by preserving the blood supply to the pancreas until the resection dissection is completed.

DOI: 10.1201/9781003341741-7

The procedure begins with a transverse or midline incision, depending on the patient, followed by a Kocher maneuver to mobilize the duodenum and the pancreatic head until the left renal vein and superior mesenteric artery are clearly visible. The portal triad is identified, and the gastroduodenal artery is dissected and clamped. The short gastric vessels are divided, and the spleen is mobilized by dividing the spleno-renal and spleno-colic ligaments. The spleen, along with the tail and body of the pancreas, is mobilized medially to the level of the superior mesenteric vein. The splenic artery and vein are then dissected, with the splenic artery being identified and looped on the superior edge of the pancreas. The splenic vein is looped distally to the entry of the inferior mesenteric vein. The duodenum is transected 3 cm distal to the pylorus using a stapler. The right gastric and gastro-epiploic blood vessels are preserved, and the stomach is reflected upwards and laterally to expose the head and body of the pancreas. The distal duodenum and proximal jejunum are transected at the ligament of Treitz. The pancreatic neck is elevated off the portal vein, and the bile duct is identified and transected at the superior border of the pancreas, with careful examination for any accessory right hepatic artery arising from the superior mesenteric artery.

The vascular structures are divided in the following order: gastroduodenal artery, splenic artery, and splenic vein. The pancreas is then placed in a cold sterile preservation solution and transported to the isolation laboratory.

In the isolation technique, various enzyme mixtures, including collagenase and protease, are used for islet cell processing. The patient receives 70 IU/kg of heparin, which circulates for 3 minutes. The islet product also contains 30 IU/kg of heparin. The patient is started on dextran at a rate of 0.5 cc per kg to a maximum of 10 cc per hour continuous infusion. Dextran inhibits the extrinsic pathway of coagulation.

The islet infusion into the portal vein system is performed by gravity. Baseline portal pressure is recorded, and pressure measurements are taken every 3 minutes. If the pressure increases to greater than 25 cm of saline, the infusion is paused for 15 minutes, and the pressure is measured again. Monitoring pressure changes at 3-minute intervals is crucial. If the pressure is less than 25 cm of saline, the infusion is restarted. If the pressure remains higher than 25 cm of saline after 15 minutes or if the total tissue volume reaches 0.25/kg, the portal infusion is stopped, and the remaining islet preparation is implanted in the peritoneal cavity as a thin film.

Islet cell allotransplantation involves isolating islet cells from a deceased-donor pancreas and subsequently transplanting them into the recipient's liver. This procedure encompasses islet isolation, processing, and subsequent implantation in the portal vein.

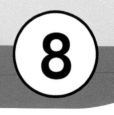

8 Small bowel transplantation

8.1 INTESTINAL FAILURE

Intestinal failure refers to the inability of a patient to meet their nutritional needs through enteral intake. This condition is considered irreversible when the patient requires ongoing parenteral nutrition (PN). The survival rates of patients on home PN are quite promising, with a 90% survival rate at 1 year, but the rates decline to 65% at 5 years. However, this treatment approach comes with its share of complications, including catheter-related sepsis, venous thrombosis, and intestinal failure-associated liver disease (IFALD).

IFALD affects more than half of the patients on long-term PN, and interestingly, it may even develop before the initiation of PN in severely malnourished patients. In children, IFALD is frequently caused by cholestasis, whereas in adults, it is commonly associated with steatohepatitis. The latter is likely due to the combination of high glucose intake, which stimulates insulin production and promotes lipogenesis, along with high lipid infusions. Both groups of patients with IFALD may experience disease progression leading to fibrosis and cirrhosis. Additionally, biliary sludge and gallstones are common in both age groups and are associated with short bowel syndrome when PN is not utilized.

For patients with intestinal failure who do not respond well to other treatments, intestinal transplantation becomes an option. However, the outcomes of this procedure vary and are better in centers with high-volume transplantation programs, in younger recipients, and in patients transplanted from home rather than those who were already inpatients. Generally, graft survival rates are approximately 80%, and patient survival rates are around 90% at 1-year post-transplant.

8.2 INDICATIONS OF TRANSPLANTATION

In pediatric patients, the aetiology of intestinal failure can be categorized into five groups. The first group comprises cases of short bowel syndrome, commonly resulting from conditions such as gastroschisis, midgut volvulus, necrotizing enterocolitis, and intestinal atresia. The second group involves motility disorders, which include long-segment Hirschsprung disease and chronic intestinal pseudo-obstruction. The third group consists of epithelial disorders characterized

DOI: 10.1201/9781003341741-8

by intractable diarrhoea, such as microvillous inclusion disease and tufting enteropathy. The fourth group includes children with a failed intestinal transplant. Lastly, the fifth group encompasses miscellaneous causes including tumours.

Intestinal transplantation is indicated for one of three main reasons:

1. Complications of parenteral nutrition
   a. PN induced liver injury
   b. Thrombosis of two or more central veins
   c. Two or more episodes of catheter-related sepsis per year requiring hospitalization
   d. A single episode of fungal catheter-related sepsis; septic shock
   e. Frequent severe dehydration due to gut losses despite intravenous fluid supplementation and PN

2. Requirement for major gut resection for tumour, such as a desmoid tumour invading the mesentery

3. Unacceptable quality of life on PN

PN, including home PN, serves as the primary treatment for pediatric patients with intestinal failure, enabling satisfactory growth and an acceptable quality of life for most individuals, although not reaching normal levels. Nonetheless, PN can lead to life-threatening complications, predominantly line sepsis, venous access loss due to thrombosis, and liver disease that may progress to cirrhosis. In severe cases, intestinal transplantation becomes the only lifesaving option. Depending on the specific underlying condition and PN-related complications, additional organ transplantation may be necessary, such as liver transplantation for patients with cirrhosis, stomach and duodenum with pancreas transplantation for those with extended motility disorders, and kidney transplantation for patients with renal failure.

The management of children with intestinal failure requires a comprehensive, multidisciplinary approach that extends throughout their lifetime. The disease typically originates in the neonatal period and necessitates initial surgical intervention. Future operations should be considered at each surgical procedure, as additional interventions may become necessary. Proper administration of PN and prevention of line infections significantly influence the long-term prognosis of children with intestinal failure.

Early contact with a specialized team in managing pediatric patients with intestinal failure is recommended if long-term PN dependency is anticipated. This early contact helps optimize the overall management of the child, allowing for the adaptation of long-term PN and preparation for potential future medical and surgical interventions, which may include nontransplant surgery or transplantation. Therefore, contacting the intestinal failure team at an early stage, particularly for children projected to require more than 50% of PN at 3 months after PN initiation, is essential to ensure the best possible outcomes and quality of life for these patients.

8.3 ASSESSMENT FOR TRANSPLANTATION

Candidates for intestinal transplantation (IT) typically present with a complex medical history and may have undergone multiple prior operations. An extensive and detailed work-up is essential to precisely evaluate the extent of intestinal failure (IF) and its potential reversibility. This work-up includes assessing the patient's history of PN and central-line complications, such as the number of catheters used, episodes of line sepsis, and the specific bacteria involved, including antibiotic resistance profiles.

Additionally, evaluating thrombotic complications and the status of patent vascular access is crucial. The presence of intestinal failure-associated liver disease (IFALD) is carefully examined, assessing for liver fibrosis or cirrhosis, jaundice, ascites, and signs of portal hypertension, such as oesophageal, gastric, or peristomal varices, and thrombocytopenia. Liver insufficiency is also considered during this assessment.

The surgical status of the abdomen, including any previous operations, and the length and function of the remaining bowel and stomas are thoroughly examined. Functionality of other organs, especially the heart, lungs, and kidneys, is also taken into account. Neurologic development and potential impairment are assessed to understand the patient's neurological status.

Serologic status and immunizations are evaluated, including the presence of anti-HLA antibodies. A sociofamilial and psychological assessment is conducted to determine the family's ability to manage the child before and after transplantation, as this support is critical for the patient's well-being.

This comprehensive evaluation process helps identify suitable candidates for intestinal transplantation, ensuring that those selected have the best chance of successful outcomes and improved quality of life post-transplantation.

The main aspects for the assessment of intestinal transplantation are the following:

1. Fitness for surgery
   a. Full cardiological and respiratory assessments
   b. Nuclear medicine glomerular filtration rate to evaluate the need of simultaneous kidney transplant
   c. Extensive venous mapping to identify perioperative access
   d. Immunization scheme and evaluate the need for splenectomy (consider meningococcal, pneumococcal, and *Haemophilus influenza* vaccine)
   e. Psychological assessment is required; assess quality of life

2. Liver disease

    a. Doppler
    b. Liver biopsy if considered
    c. Fibroscan

3. Surgical anatomy

    a. Careful scan and contrast imaging of the remaining bowel, together with endoscopic inspection of any bowel to be left in situ to exclude disease, and also inspection of any bowel to be removed to confirm the diagnosis if required

8.4 DONORS

Typically, deceased donors are the preferred source for intestinal transplants, although there have been some reported cases of living-related donations for isolated small bowel transplants. Ensuring the appropriate size of the graft is crucial and depends on various factors, such as the donor to recipient weight ratio, the native organs that have been removed, the type of graft being implanted, and whether the recipient's abdominal cavity is small (for short bowel intestinal transplantation) or distended (for intestinal motility disorders with chronic intestinal dilatation).

8.5 TYPES OF TRANSPLANT

A diverse range of grafts can be performed, all aimed at providing enough length of small intestine to enable the recipient to be free from parenteral nutrition dependence. The inclusion of the large intestine in the transplant helps reduce fluid losses. To facilitate biopsy, the terminal ileum is brought out as an ileostomy, but this may be reversed in the future to restore gut continuity. In cases of pre-existing renal failure, simultaneous consideration for a kidney transplant is recommended.

8.6 ISOLATED SMALL BOWEL

An isolated intestinal transplant, which may include small bowel with or without the right colon, is specifically recommended for patients with IF who have normal motility in the stomach and duodenum and do not exhibit significant liver disease. In this type of transplant, the native stomach, duodenum, pancreas, spleen, and liver are preserved (see Figure 8.1).

    The surgical procedure involves carefully anastomosing the superior mesenteric artery of the graft to the recipient's infrarenal aorta, and the mesentericoportal

Isolated Small Bowel

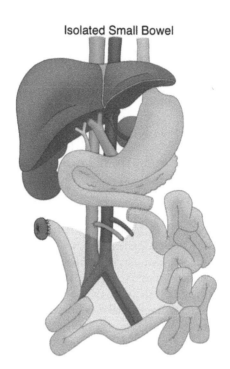

Figure 8.1 Isolated small bowel transplant.

axis of the graft vein is joined to the infrarenal vena cava. Furthermore, the proximal jejunum of the graft is connected to the native jejunum.

One of the significant advantages of an isolated intestinal transplant is that it allows for the potential removal of the graft if serious complications arise. In such cases, the patient can be safely returned to PN until they are fit for a possible retransplant. This flexibility ensures the well-being of the patient and allows for a contingency plan should any complications arise during the post-transplant period.

8.7 COMBINED LIVER AND INTESTINAL TRANSPLANTATION

This type of transplant is a multiorgan graft that includes the liver, pancreas, duodenum, small bowel, and may or may not include the right colon. It is specifically indicated for patients with IF who have normal motility in the stomach and duodenum but present with significant liver disease. In this procedure, the native liver is removed, and a portocaval anastomosis is created between the native portal vein and vena cava.

While the native stomach, duodenum, pancreas, and spleen are preserved, the arterial axis of the graft, including the celiac trunk and superior mesenteric artery, is meticulously connected to the recipient's infrarenal aorta. For venous drainage, the suprahepatic vena cava of the graft is joined to the native suprahepatic vena cava in a "piggyback" fashion, ensuring proper blood flow and graft functionality.

To facilitate the procedure, the first portion of the duodenum of the graft is closed, and the graft jejunum is connected to the native jejunum using a Roux loop technique. This anastomosis helps maintain the continuity of the digestive tract and allows for the proper flow of ingested food.

This multiorgan graft offers a comprehensive solution for patients with intestinal failure and significant liver disease. By combining the liver, pancreas, duodenum, small bowel, and potentially the right colon in one transplant, it addresses both intestinal and hepatic issues, providing the patient with a chance for improved gut function and metabolic stability. The preservation of specific native organs further enhances the success and compatibility of the graft, ensuring optimal outcomes for the recipient.

8.8 MULTIVISCERAL TRANSPLANT

This type of transplant involves a comprehensive combination of organs, including the liver, stomach, duodenum, pancreas, small bowel, and may or may not include the right colon and kidney(s) (Figure 8.2). It is specifically indicated for patients with intestinal failure (IF) who have impaired motility in the stomach and duodenum, such as those with pan-intestinal Hirschsprung disease and chronic intestinal pseudo-obstruction, and significant liver disease.

This transplant becomes necessary when there is a need for en-bloc ablation of the native organs, including the liver, pancreas, duodenum, and intestine. Such a situation may arise due to previous surgeries and portal hypertension, which make selective dissection of native abdominal organs impractical. In rare cases, it might also be required because of the presence of a tumour.

For patients with intestinal failure and severe associated liver disease, the transplant would include both the liver and small bowel. This is typically achieved by implanting a segment of the stomach, duodenum, and pancreas, which receives its arterial supply from the coeliac trunk and superior mesenteric artery. The venous drainage is facilitated through the hepatic veins.

During the transplant procedure, the donor stomach is anastomosed to a cuff of the recipient's stomach just below the diaphragmatic hiatus. To prevent gastric emptying, the transplanted stomach is denervated, resulting in the closure of the pylorus. To address this, a gastric drainage procedure is necessary, which can involve either a pyloroplasty or gastrojejunostomy.

This complex transplant approach provides a comprehensive solution for patients with intestinal failure and impaired motility in the stomach and duodenum, along with significant liver disease. By combining multiple organs, it

Multivisceral

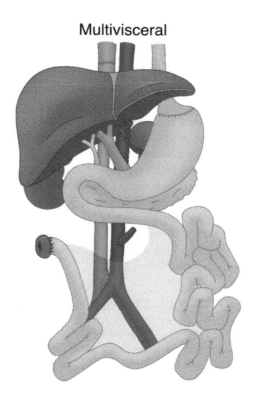

Figure 8.2 Multivisceral transplant.

addresses the underlying issues effectively and offers a chance for improved gut function and metabolic stability. The surgical techniques utilized in this procedure are carefully tailored to ensure proper organ integration and functional outcomes for the recipient.

This transplant procedure involves the transplantation of the stomach, pancreas, and duodenum, along with the small bowel, and optionally the right colon. It is typically indicated for patients with IF who have impaired motility of their native stomach and duodenum, such as those with pan-intestinal Hirschsprung disease and chronic intestinal pseudo-obstruction, but without significant liver disease. In cases where the liver is only minimally diseased and there is a possibility of recovery, a transplant excluding the liver is considered appropriate.

When there is a history of gastric or pancreatic disease, such as pancreatitis related to PN, the bowel segment for transplantation should include the stomach and duodenum. The portal vein of the graft is then anastomosed to the recipient portal vein at the hilum of the liver.

During the procedure, the upper part of the native stomach, duodenum, pancreas, spleen, and liver are preserved. The arterial axis of the graft, comprising the

Modified Multivisceral

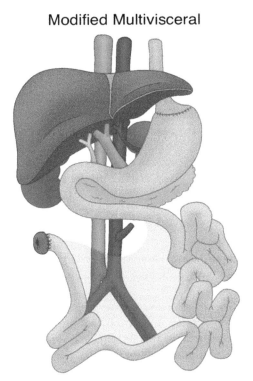

Figure 8.3 Modified multivisceral transplant.

celiac trunk and superior mesenteric artery, is connected to the recipient infrarenal aorta. The mesentericoportal axis of the graft is joined to the recipient infrarenal vena cava.

To facilitate functional continuity, the native and transplanted hemi-stomachs are connected. The native first portion of the duodenum is closed, and the native jejunum is connected to the transplanted jejunum in the form of a Roux loop.

This transplant approach is designed to address the specific needs of patients with impaired motility of the stomach and duodenum without significant liver disease. By carefully preserving essential organs and ensuring proper graft integration, this procedure offers a chance for improved gut function and quality of life for the recipient. The selection of appropriate graft components is based on the patient's medical history, liver condition, and the anticipated outcomes following transplantation (Figure 8.3).

In all cases, a distal ileostomy is performed to provide easy access to the graft for intestinal biopsies and endoscopies. When the right colon is transplanted, its distal end is either anastomosed to the native rectum (patients with short gut or mucosal diseases) or a temporary distal colostomy is created (Hirschsprung disease). Cholecystectomy and gastrostomy are generally performed if not done previously.

8.9 POST-TRANSPLANT CARE

After undergoing intestinal transplantation, the resumption of intestinal transit is usually rapid, allowing for the gradual introduction of enteral feeding within 2 to 7 days following the surgery. The graft's denervation contributes to the accelerated transit time, facilitating the transition to enteral feeding. During the early stages of recovery, close monitoring is essential to rule out any dysfunction of the graft, such as rejection or infection, which could potentially interfere with the feeding process.

Once graft-related issues have been ruled out, healthcare providers may consider the use of antimotility agents, such as loperamide or codeine, to help regulate intestinal motility. These medications can effectively slow down the transit time and promote the proper absorption of nutrients, ensuring adequate nourishment for the patient.

In cases where the postoperative course progresses without complications, patients can expect to achieve full enteral feeding within approximately one month after the transplantation. This timeline may vary depending on the individual's response to treatment, overall health condition, and the successful adaptation of the transplanted intestine.

Throughout the recovery period, the nutrition team plays a crucial role in monitoring the patient's nutritional status, adjusting feeding plans as needed, and providing personalized dietary recommendations. Close collaboration between the nutritionists, physicians, and the entire healthcare team is essential to optimize the patient's nutritional intake and promote a successful recovery.

For some patients, achieving full enteral feeding within a month represents a significant milestone on the road to recovery and improved quality of life. The ability to transition from parenteral nutrition to enteral feeding signifies successful graft adaptation and functional restoration of the intestinal tract.

It is important to note that each patient's recovery is unique, and individual responses to transplantation may vary. Therefore, a comprehensive and tailored nutrition plan, along with diligent follow-up care, ensures that patients receive the best possible support during their post-transplant journey towards optimal nutritional health.

8.10 PERIOPERATIVE COMPLICATIONS

Various surgical complications can arise after intestinal transplantation, including obstructions, peritonitis, fistulas, and pancreatitis. Detecting these complications can be challenging, especially in patients undergoing steroid therapy, which can mask symptoms.

Vascular monitoring of the graft is crucial, and observation of the stoma's colour provides important clues about its perfusion. Additionally, in cases where the graft includes the liver, regular ultrasounds should be conducted to assess the vascular health of the transplant.

One significant risk is the possibility of thrombosis in the arterial supply or venous drainage of the graft. This risk is heightened in recipients who have experienced the loss of their original bowel due to a procoagulant tendency. However, in some cases, liver replacement may have resolved this issue, reducing the risk of thrombosis.

Another common challenge faced during the recovery period is the delayed resumption of normal bowel function. The stomach is often the last organ to regain normal peristalsis and emptying, which can take more than 3 weeks after the transplantation. To ensure adequate nutrition during this time, patients may receive nutrients through a jejunostomy into the new bowel.

The post-operative care of intestinal transplant recipients requires careful monitoring and prompt management of any complications that may arise. Early detection of surgical issues and vigilant vascular monitoring can contribute significantly to the patient's recovery and overall success of the transplant. Nutritional support during the recovery period plays a crucial role in helping patients regain their strength and improve their quality of life following intestinal transplantation. As each patient's recovery process is unique, individualized care and close follow-up with the medical team are essential to achieving the best possible outcomes and ensuring long-term graft function and recipient well-being.

8.11 TRANSPLANT-RELATED COMPLICATIONS

Various surgical complications can arise after intestinal transplantation, including obstructions, peritonitis, fistulas, and pancreatitis. Detecting these complications can be challenging, especially in patients undergoing steroid therapy, which can mask symptoms.

Vascular monitoring of the graft is crucial, and observation of the stoma's colour provides important clues about its perfusion. Additionally, in cases where the graft includes the liver, regular ultrasounds should be conducted to assess the vascular health of the transplant.

One significant risk is the possibility of thrombosis in the arterial supply or venous drainage of the graft. This risk is heightened in recipients who have experienced the loss of their original bowel due to a procoagulant tendency. However, in some cases, liver replacement may have resolved this issue, reducing the risk of thrombosis.

Another common challenge faced during the recovery period is the delayed resumption of normal bowel function. The stomach is often the last organ to regain normal peristalsis and emptying, which can take more than 3 weeks after the transplantation. To ensure adequate nutrition during this time, patients may receive nutrients through a jejunostomy into the new bowel.

The postoperative care of intestinal transplant recipients requires careful monitoring and prompt management of any complications that may arise. Early detection of surgical issues and vigilant vascular monitoring can contribute significantly to the patient's recovery and overall success of the transplant. Nutritional support during the recovery period plays a crucial role in helping patients regain their strength and improve their quality of life following intestinal transplantation. As each patient's recovery process is unique, individualized care and close follow-up with the medical team are essential to achieving the best possible outcomes and ensuring long-term graft function and recipient well-being.

8.12 OUTCOMES

Over the years, the short-term outcomes of intestinal transplantation have shown significant improvement, reflecting the growing experience in this field. Currently, the 1-year patient and graft survival rates are promising, with isolated bowel recipients achieving 89% and 79%, respectively, and liver-intestine recipients achieving 72% and 69%, respectively.

However, the medium-term results still present challenges, as the patient and graft survival rates decrease to 46% and 29%, respectively, for isolated bowel recipients, and 42% and 39%, respectively, for liver-intestine recipients at the 10-year mark. Data from the International Intestine Transplant Registry, spanning from 1985 to 2003 and including 989 grafts in 923 patients, shed light on the causes of death after transplantation. Sepsis was the most common cause (46%), followed by graft rejection (11.2%), post-transplant lymphomas (6.2%), and other factors such as graft thrombosis, respiratory causes, technical issues, and multiorgan failure.

Nonetheless, recent decades have seen noteworthy advancements that have contributed to improved outcomes. Better patient preparation and optimal timing for transplantation, advances in surgical techniques, availability of new and more effective immunosuppressive drugs and regimens, and enhanced monitoring and management of postoperative complications have all played a role in the enhanced results.

Despite these improvements, the shortage of suitable grafts remains a significant challenge, and patients continue to face the risk of mortality while waiting for a suitable match. The ongoing efforts to enhance outcomes, especially in the long term, hold the potential to transform intestinal transplantation from solely a lifesaving procedure to one that significantly improves the quality of life for recipients. Moreover, the economic advantages of transplantation over long-term parenteral nutrition may further solidify its position as a valuable treatment option for eligible patients. With continuous research and progress, the field of intestinal transplantation is expected to witness even more positive developments in the future.

9 Immunosuppression

An implanted donor organ is recognized as a non-self by the recipient's immune system and triggers mechanisms aiming at its destruction, i.e., rejection. Mitigating the immune response to the graft prolongs its survival. It is achieved by a combination of medications targeting different components of the immune response. These therapies put transplant recipients at increased risk of infections and developing specific forms of cancer. There is ongoing research in minimizing immunosuppression and inducing tolerance to the transplanted organ.

9.1 TYPES OF REJECTION

Rejection is an immunological process initiated by an encounter with the grafted non-self tissue and executed by interplay of innate and acquired immunological responses. It is mediated by immune cells and their products. Antigen-presenting cells, T and B lymphocytes, interact via their receptors and initiate the destruction of the graft by cytotoxic cells, protein complexes, and antibodies.

Proteins expressed on the donor cells that are capable of stimulating alloimmunity and antibody production are referred to as alloantigens. These antigens usually belong to Major Histocompatibility Complex (MHC) molecules that are hugely polymorphic, generating almost a unique pattern for an individual. They are called Human Leukocyte Antigens (HLA) and are the base for compatibility matching. A better match means more similarities between the HLA pattern of the donor and recipient. ABO antigens are expressed on the endothelial cells of the implanted organ and, therefore, can become a target for antibodies if the donor and recipient are blood group incompatible. Antibody-mediated cell damage often involves activating a system of enzymatic proteins named complement cascade. Histological staining for complement components of the graft biopsy is an adjunct to histological diagnosis of the rejection.

Rejection is broadly divided into its timing (hyper-acute, acute, and chronic) and the type of immune mechanisms that predominate (T-cell or antibody mediated). There is extensive literature on this topic, and for the purpose of this book, it has been simplified with a focus on the rationale behind therapeutic protocols. This chapter will provide an overview of the mechanisms of action of

DOI: 10.1201/9781003341741-9

immunosuppressants in clinical use in pediatric transplantation and basis for immunological monitoring.

Hyperacute rejection is graft destruction seen soon after reperfusion of the graft due to pre-formed antibodies against blood group antigens. If the recipient's immune system encountered non-self HLA previously (pregnancy, blood transfusion, transplant), circulating anti-HLA antibodies might be another cause.

Acute rejection is either T-cell or antibody mediated, or a combination of both.

Chronic rejection is usually slowly ongoing organ damage due to low levels of donor-specific anti-HLA antibodies (DSA).

The liver is an organ less easily damaged by immunological processes than the kidneys. Therefore, immunosuppression protocols differ, but it is now recognized that antibody-mediated rejection happens in liver grafts, and it should be promptly diagnosed and treated. In kidney transplantation, the intensity of immunosuppression is stratified based on immunological risks. In pancreas transplantation, immunosuppression usually matches that of kidney recipients with a high immunological risk.

Hyperacute rejection is avoided by performing a crossmatch test between recipient serum and donor leukocytes. If pre-formed antibodies against the allograft are present, they will damage donor cells. This can be verified by microscope (cytotoxic crossmatch) or fluorescence (flow crossmatch). Most organ transplantation protocols include intensified immunosuppression at implantation and life-long maintenance immunosuppression. Induction immunosuppression is to combat early rejection. Maintenance immunosuppression is to prevent further rejection episodes and de novo formation of DSA. Additional tests should guide the most appropriate treatment if rejection results in allograft injury.

9.2 INDUCTION IMMUNOSUPPRESSION

Steroids are generously used at induction and then usually gradually withdrawn. They are anti-inflammatory and have a broad spectrum of action resulting in diverse side effects. The acceleration of hepatitis C virus (HCV) infection is a major concern. A quick tapper of steroids and steroid-free regimens reduces the incidence of fibrosis related to HCV reinfection and HCV recurrence.

Lymphodepleting protocols comprise polyclonal or monoclonal antibodies (mAb) against lymphocytes, such as anti-thymocyte globulin (ATG) or alemtuzumab (anti-CD52 cytolytic antibody). Basiliximab is a monoclonal antibody blocking the receptor for Interleukin-2 and preventing clonal expansion of lymphocytes. This agent is used in low and intermediate immunological risks kidney transplants and liver transplants requiring delayed initiation of calcineurin inhibitor due to renal impairment.

9.3 MAINTENANCE IMMUNOSUPPRESSION

Maintenance immunosuppression is with a combination of two to three medications targeting different arms of the immune response toward allograft.

Calcineurin inhibitors (CIN), such as cyclosporine and tacrolimus, stop signal transduction from T-cell receptor to the nucleus and further gene activation, suppressing T-cell activation and cytokine production.

Sirolimus and everolimus (hydroxyethyl derivative of sirolimus) inhibit mTOR (mechanistic target of rapamycin – serine/threonine-specific protein kinase); mTOR regulates cellular metabolism, growth, and proliferation.

Azathioprine and mycophenolic acid (MPA) are antimetabolites that affect proliferation. Mycophenolate mofetil (MMF) and mycophenolate sodium (Myfortic) are converted to MPA. MPA inhibits inosine monophosphate dehydrogenase preventing the formation of GMP. Cells depleted of GMP cannot synthesize GTP or d-GTP and, therefore, cannot replicate. Azathioprine is a pro-drug of 6-mercaptopurine (6-MP) 6-MP is a false substrate that inhibits purine synthesis and thus interferes with RNA and DNA synthesis. Steroids interfere with the transcription of multiple genes involved in inflammation. They bind with cytoplasmatic receptors and interact with glucocorticoid response elements in various gene promote sequences that regulate gene expressions.

The effect of steroids on bone metabolism and growth is of particular concern in pediatric recipients. Steroid-free maintenance immunosuppression should be attempted unless other circumstances, such as high immunological risk or frequent rejection episodes.

CIN-related toxicity requires reducing the dose of the causative agent. Switching to belatacept is another option. Belatacept is a monoclonal antibody blocking CTLA-4, a molecule involved in T-cell activation.

Specific infection complications also require modification of immunosuppression, although there is always a balance between putting a patient at risk for rejection (see Table 9.1).

9.4 KIDNEY TRANSPLANTATION

Immunosuppressive strategies in pediatric recipients are consistent with adult protocols adjusted for the abovementioned considerations. There are, however, significant differences between countries in preferences for antibody-based induction therapy. In North America, lymphocyte depletion with anti-thymocyte

Table 9.1 **Basic Immunosuppressants**

AGENT	MECHANISM	SIDE EFFECTS
Steroids	Anti-inflammatory	• Diabetes • Fluid retention and hypertension • Emotional liability • Hyperlipidaemia • Poor wound healing • Adrenal suppression • Increase in hepatitis C virus replication
Cyclosporine	Inhibits IL-2 and Interferon-gamma production	• Renal toxicity • Hypertension and hyperlipidaemia • Hyperkalaemia and hypomagnesaemia • Neurotoxicity: altered mental status, polyneuropathy, myoclonus, seizures, hallucinations • Gingival hyperplasia, hirsutism
Tacrolimus	Inhibits IL-2 and Interferon-gamma production	• Hyperglycaemia and diabetes • Hyperkalaemia and hypomagnesaemia • Nephrotoxicity • Neurotoxicity: tremor and seizures • Neuropsychiatric problems: confusion, loss of appetite, insomnia, depression, vivid nightmares • PRES (posterior reversible encephalopathy syndrome) • Alopecia
Sirolimus	mTOR inhibitor	• Delayed wound healing
Everolimus	mTOR inhibitor	• Stomatitis and loss of taste • Leukopenia and anaemia
Azathioprine	inhibits purine synthesis	• Bone marrow suppression • Nausea, vomiting • Pancreatitis and hepatotoxicity
MMF	Inhibits GMP synthesis	• Bone marrow suppression • Gastrointestinal complaints: abdominal pain, • Ileus, nausea, vomiting • Oral ulceration
Myfortic	Inhibits GMP synthesis	• Similar to MMF but less gastrointestinal disturbances

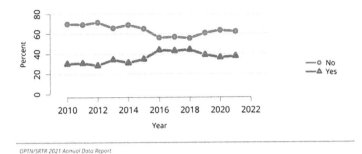

Figure 9.1 Induction agent use in pediatric kidney transplant recipients. (From OPTN/SRTR 2019 Annual Data Report: Kidney. Hart A, et al. JJ. Am J Transplant. 2021 Feb;21 Suppl 2:21–137.)

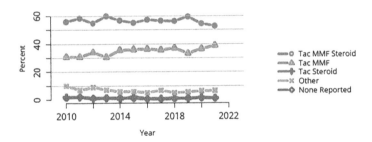

Figure 9.2 Immunosuppression regimen use in pediatric kidney transplant recipients. (From OPTN/SRTR 2019 Annual Data Report: Kidney. Hart A, et al. JJ Am J Transplant. 2021 Feb;21 Suppl 2:21–137.)

Tac = tacrolimus, MMF = all mycophenolateagents.

globulin is a common practice. As a result, ATG is used at induction in one-quarter of children transplanted in the United States. In the United Kingdom, alemtuzumab is administered to patients undergoing renal transplants stratified as a high-immunological risk. This is rarely the case in pediatric recipients. Children usually receive basiliximab on the day of their transplant and 4 days after.

The majority of children are on triple maintenance immunosuppression with tacrolimus, mycophenolate mofetil, and prednisolone. An increasing percentage of children are no longer receiving chronic steroids.

In 2021, almost all (94%) pediatric kidney transplant recipients in the United States had some form of induction (Figure 9.1). The most common maintenance immunosuppression regimens at hospital discharge were tacrolimus, MMF, and steroids in 52.7% of recipients, followed by tacrolimus and MMF in 38.8% (Figure 9.2).

9.5 ABO-INCOMPATIBLE KIDNEY TRANSPLANTATION

ABO-incompatible (ABOi) kidney transplantation is an effective strategy for increasing the pool of potential living donors for patients without a suitable compatible donor. It requires pre-transplant removal of antibodies and B-cell depletion and monitoring of anti-ABO titers in the perioperative period. Good long-term outcomes are comparable with compatible transplants.

Historically, desensitization strategies have relied on splenectomy and plasmapheresis. A combination of B-cell depletion with rituximab, antibody removal with immunoadsorption or plasmapheresis, and triple maintenance immunosuppression, including calcineurin inhibitor (tacrolimus), an antiproliferative agent (mycophenolate mofetil), and steroids are currently being used in London, UK. A tailored desensitization protocol without routine postoperative antibody removal allows minimizing desensitization in low titer patients.

The approach is based on the baseline anti-ABO titers. All patients with titers of 1 in 8 or more receive rituximab (375 mg/m^2) one month before transplant and Basiliximab on days 0 and 4. Patients with titers 1 in 64 or more undergo Immunoadsorption (IA), whereas those with titers of 1 in 32 or 1 in 16 are treated with double filtration plasmapheresis (DFPP). The aim is to reduce the titers to 1 in 8 or less at the time of transplant. Antibody removal is performed on consecutive days before the transplant. A fall of 2 dilutions in the titers with each session of DFPP/IA is expected. Patients with titers of 1 in 8 receive rituximab with no antibody removal. Those with titers of less than 1 in 8 receive Basiliximab without Rituximab or antibody removal. Triple maintenance immunosuppression is used in all patients with tacrolimus and mycophenolate mofetil starting one week before the surgery and steroids on the day of the operation (see Figure 9.3).

9.5.1 HLA-INCOMPATIBLE KIDNEY TRANSPLANTATION

HLA-incompatible (HLAi) kidney transplantation is an option for highly sensitized patients with low chances of compatible transplants. Highly sensitized patients have multiple anti-HLA antibodies with a high probability of positive crossmatch with potential donors. In the UK, the level of sensitization is derived from the proportion of the last ten thousand deceased donors to whom that patient has antibodies. Highly sensitized patients have calculated Reaction Frequency (cRF) > 85% (they would be HLA incompatible with 8,500 donors out of 10,000). Similarly, in the US, the PRA (panel reactive antibody) is calculated from HLA typed donor population and the patient's anti-HLA antibodies specificities detected. It used to be determined by testing the patient's serum against a panel of HLA-typed donor cells and estimating the likelihood of finding a crossmatch compatible donor.

Highly sensitized children are unlikely to receive kidneys via national living donor kidney sharing schemes as they are usually sensitized to common HLA

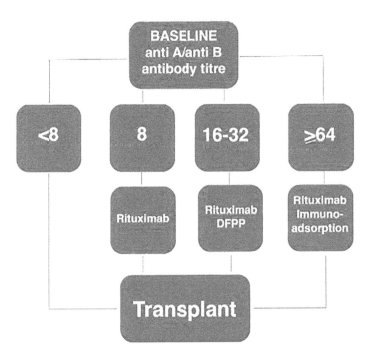

Figure 9.3 Flow chart showing immune desensitization strategy for ABOi renal transplant. (From Immune Desensitization Allows Pediatric Blood Group Incompatible Kidney Transplantation. Stojanovic J, et al. Transplantation. 2017 Jun;101(6):1242–124.)

antigens. Desensitization aims to remove a sufficient amount of antibodies to ensure a lack of reactivity of recipient serum to donor tissue at the time of transplant (negative crossmatch) with one of the available techniques: plasma exchange, double filtration plasmapheresis, immunoadsorption.

Outcomes of HLAi renal transplants are inferior to compatible ones, associated with increased morbidity from desensitization, and carry increased risks of rejection. The decision to proceed with HLAi in a child should not be taken lightly.

In countries with well-developed deceased donation programs, it has been recognized that highly sensitized patients end up waiting years for an appropriate donor offer, and current allocation policies prioritize them (see Figure 9.4).

9.6 LIVER TRANSPLANTATION

Induction immunosuppression in liver transplantation facilitates the minimization of steroids and reduces exposure to calcineurin inhibitors rather than augmenting overall immunosuppression. In the United States, one-third of pediatric

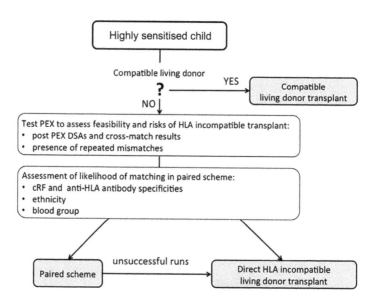

Figure 9.4 Algorithm supporting decision-making process as to whether to consider HLA-incompatible renal transplantation in a child. (From Desensitiation Protocol Enabling Pediatric Crossmatch-Positive Renal Transplantation: Successful HLA-Antibody-Incompatible Renal Transplantation of Two Highly Sensitized Children. Adamusiak AM et al. Pediatr Nephrol. 2017 Feb;32(2):359–364. doi:10.1007/s00467-016-3489-z.)

PEX = plasma exchange, DSAs = donor-specific antibodies, cRF = calculated reaction frequency.

liver transplants in children have induction immunosuppression administrated. The preferred choice has been Basiliximab over ATG.

Maintenance immunosuppression regimens usually comprise tacrolimus. In randomized control trials, tacrolimus proved superior to cyclosporine with significantly lower rates of acute and chronic rejection, albeit with no improvement in patient or graft survival. Mycophenolate mofetil has largely replaced azathioprine as the anti-metabolite of choice. With the widespread use of tacrolimus, with or without mycophenolate, there has been substantial interest in exploring corticosteroid minimization or avoidance strategies. Clinical trials showed that recipients in the steroid-free regimen had superior one-year rejection-free survival and significant linear growth. Additional studies have confirmed that Basiliximab supported complete steroid elimination with a significantly lower incidence of acute rejection, overall infection, or viral infection. Currently, in the United States, approximately 20% of children undergo liver transplantation with complete steroid avoidance, and one year after transplantation, 40% of pediatric liver transplant recipients remain on corticosteroids.

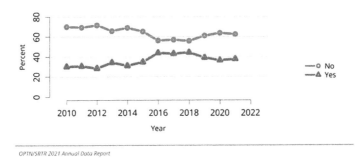

OPTN/SRTR 2021 Annual Data Report

Figure 9.5 Induction agent use in pediatric liver transplant recipients. (From OPTN/SRTR 2021 Annual Data Report: Liver. Kwong AJ, et al. Am J Transplant. 2023 Feb;23(2 Suppl 1):S178–S263.)

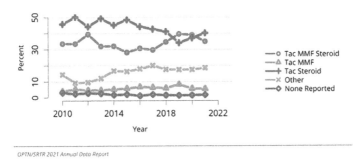

OPTN/SRTR 2021 Annual Data Report

Figure 9.6 Immunosuppression regimen use in pediatric liver transplant recipients. (From OPTN/SRTR 2021 Annual Data Report: Liver. Kwong AJ, et al. Am J Transplant. 2023 Feb;23(2 Suppl 1):S178–S263.)

Tac = tacrolimus. MMF = all mycophenolate agents.

In 2021, 62.3% of pediatric liver transplant recipients in the United States received no induction therapy (Figure 9.5). The most common initial immunosuppression regimens were tacrolimus and steroids (39.9%), followed by tacrolimus, mycophenolate agent, and steroids (34.7%) (Figure 9.6).

9.7 ABO INCOMPATIBLE LIVER TRANSPLANTATION

Techniques of antibody removal and B-cell depleting agents can facilitate performing liver transplants across the ABO barrier. Although in this kind of transplant, immunosuppression and rejection surveillance are intensified, the property of the liver being able to resist recipient antibodies allows proceeding with them even in the deceased donor setting with urgent indication and non-compatible donor available.

9.8 POST-TRANSPLANT MONITORING AND DIAGNOSIS OF REJECTION

During the early postoperative period, frequent lab tests should be performed to detect deterioration in graft function early. Levels of immunosuppression medications should guide prompt dose adjustments.

Kidney rejection can be suspected when there is decreasing urine output and rising serum creatinine. Fever and graft tenderness used to be observed but with calcineurin inhibitors are now rarely seen. If present, it might be a sequel of non-compliance. The differential diagnosis includes ureteric obstruction, collections, renal vascular compromise from stenosis, and an infectious process. Urine analysis and culture should be performed to assess the possibility of infection. Ultrasound can visualise an obstruction due to collections (hematoma, lymphocele, urinoma) or ureteric stricture and provide information on blood flow velocities. On a radionuclide renal scan, rapid uptake of the tracer by the kidney and delayed excretion suggest rejection, but it does not allow for distinguishing among various causes of intragraft dysfunction (rejection vs. CIN toxicity vs. acute tubular necrosis).

Concerns for rejection should be addressed with biopsy and laboratory tests of DSA presence/levels in the patient's serum. Ultrasound-guided percutaneous renal biopsy for an extraperitoneal kidney is usually performed; an intraperitoneal graft might require computer tomography. In some circumstances, treatment of the rejection might be initiated before formal histological diagnosis.

Renal biopsy is associated with potential complications, specifically bleeding and related graft loss. Thus, there is a growing interest in non-invasive diagnostics with a laboratory assay that has been developed and is commercially available. It is based on highly sensitive monitoring of donor cells debris in recipient blood. Detection of donor-derived cell-free DNA (dd-cfDNA, AlloSure) is associated with rejection in adult kidney transplants. There are an increasing number of studies on its utility in children. Studies showed dd-cfDNA to be highly predictive of histological rejection in pediatric renal transplant recipients.

The diagnostic and therapeutic algorithms for early acute cellular rejection for pediatric liver transplant recipients parallel those for adult liver transplant recipients. Considering the increased technical difficulty and a higher rate of surgical complications for pediatric liver transplantation, an ultrasound Doppler examination is an essential first step in assessing allograft dysfunction typically manifested by elevated liver tests. First, the hepatic arterial, portal venous, or biliary complications must be ruled out, and then a liver biopsy should be obtained. The most common approach to liver biopsy is percutaneous, with ultrasound guidance. An alternative is a transjugular approach performed by an interventional radiologist.

9.9 TREATMENT OF T-CELL-MEDIATED REJECTION

The first line of treatment rejection is steroid pulses: a single daily dose of 10–20 mg/kg of methylprednisolone for 3 consecutive days.

Steroid-resistant rejection is treated with ATG. It is given in a dose of 1.5–2 mg/kg for a. total of 10–14 days, although these practices might vary between transplant centers. It might be advisable to monitor CD3 cells during treatment and restrict the frequency of dosing only to days when the count is greater than 20 cells/mm^3.

Follow-up biopsy may be necessary to assess treatment efficacy, particularly if there is suspicion of incomplete response. After treatment of an acute rejection episode, augmentation of maintenance immunosuppression is often considered.

9.10 TREATMENT OF ANTIBODY-MEDIATED REJECTION

Therapies affecting antibody production, such as anti-CD20 monoclonal antibody and intravenous immunoglobulin with immunomodulatory effects, are usually combined with a series of antibody removal procedures. The level of DSA is monitored throughout the treatment.

9.11 INDUCTION OF TOLERANCE

The initial goal of transplant immunologists joining forces with surgeons in the mid-twentieth century was to make a kidney recipient tolerant to the allograft. After it was achieved in the mice, the developed protocol was hoped to be applied in clinical practice. The treatment was with bone marrow ablation by irradiation and a bone marrow transplant followed by a kidney transplant from the same donor. After a few attempts, it was abandoned due to high mortality related to irradiation and graft-versus-host disease (GVHD). GVHD is due to lymphocytes of the donor attacking recipient cells, especially of the skin and gastrointestinal system. Instead of inducing tolerance, lifelong maintenance immunosuppression keeping the immune system under control has been wildly adopted. Immunosuppression protocols have greatly improved over decades. The combination of different agents and monitoring of drug levels help guide dose reduction, and as a result, side effects can be minimized and graft function preserved. But consequences of immunosuppression, such as infections and cancers, persist, and most allografts eventually fail. This is a reason why there are ongoing attempts to induce tolerance. These trials involved harsh pre-conditioning, and therefore children were not eligible. A few pediatric cases were reported from Stanford of recent successful combined allogeneic stem cell transplant (SCT) followed by a kidney from the same related living donor. The infusion of the stem cells was modified to reduce the magnitude of GVHD. Three patients treated with this protocol are off immunosuppression with good renal function.

It has also been realized that a subgroup of patients can maintain an excellent long-term graft function without immunosuppression. This is more common in liver recipients. No tolerance markers are yet available in clinical practice, and therefore there are no intentional attempts to stop immunosuppression in children.

9.12 MEDICATION ADHERENCE

Non-adherence is often cited as a cause of long-term graft loss in pediatric renal transplant recipients, especially adolescents. A common reason for non-adherence is the alteration in appearance that accompanies immunosuppressive medications, specifically related to daily steroid administration. Some factors, such as adolescence, poor socio-economic status, and family dynamics, have been associated with increased levels of non-adherence. Precaution measures are educational programs and family-based therapy to enhance motivation.

Infectious complications before and after pediatric liver transplantation

10

10.1 INTRODUCTION

Liver transplantation (LTX) is the only definitive and lifesaving treatment in end-stage liver disease in children. In the last few decades, the outcome of LTX in children has improved drastically with a survival of more than 90% at 5 years. The various factors that have contributed to this are; advances in surgical techniques, newer immunosuppressive agents and improved diagnostic methods for identifying and preventing infections. However, infections continue to evolve and remain the leading cause of morbidity, mortality, and hospital costs among transplant recipients. Following LTX, these young patients undergo profound immunosuppression to prevent organ rejection, making them highly susceptible to various types of infections. Infections can also contribute to allograft dysfunction. Infections pose a significant challenge in the management of pediatric liver transplant recipients (PLTR). Understanding the incidence, timing and types of infections, and associated risk factors before and after transplant is crucial for healthcare providers involved in the care of PLTR. To best manage the infectious complications, it is important to evaluate the infectious risk before transplant and donor-derived risk of infections. Herein we discuss pre-transplant infectious disease evaluation of transplant candidate and donor, immunizations and post-transplant infections alongside the preventive and management strategies for infections in PLTR.

10.2 PRE-TRANSPLANT INFECTIOUS DISEASE EVALUATION AND IMMUNIZATIONS

When a patient is evaluated for transplantation, the opportunity arises to assess the individual's risk for infection and how one may modify those risks through prophylactic and therapeutic strategies. Evaluation should be performed by an experienced transplant infectious disease specialist. Pre-transplant infectious disease evaluation focuses on exposure history, prior infections, serologic testing for latent infections, distant exposures, identifying colonization patterns of

DOI: 10.1201/9781003341741-10

multidrug-resistant organisms (MDRO), and administration of vaccines. The risk of acquiring rare infections is increasing because of greater global mobility. Additional evaluation should be considered for some endemic infectious diseases, beyond recommended standard testing for transplant candidates and donors.

10.3 ACTIVE AND LATENT INFECTIONS BEFORE TRANSPLANT

Children with end-stage liver disease are at high risk of bacterial infections. Spontaneous bacterial peritonitis (SBP) and cholangitis are serious complication in these patients and has led to long-term use of antibiotics. A drug history of multiple courses of antibiotics is particularly important because it may predispose the patient to infections with MDRO or fungal infections in the early postoperative period. All transplant candidates should be tested for active infections pre-operatively and fully treated wherever possible. In patients with active infections before transplant such as SBP and blood stream infections, transplant should be delayed where possible. However, there is no data to suggest what should be a safe interval between infection and transplantation. It is important to fully treat and investigate by repeating cultures, serology, radiography, or other tests required to diagnose the infection. This may not be practical in situations of emergency transplant or very sick patients who are offered a deceased donor organ, where management should be individualized in consultation with a microbiologist or infectious-disease consultant knowledgeable in transplant infectious diseases. It is important to detect active infections and fully treat such infections prior to transplant (see Table 10.1).

LATENT BACTERIAL INFECTIONS AND COLONIZATION

- **MDRO:** Colonization and infection with emerging MDRO is an increasing problem in patients awaiting transplantation. Pre-transplant screening should be considered based on the local transplant center's prevalence and epidemiology of MDRO. The most common MDRO include, vancomycin-resistant *Enterococcus faecium* (VRE), methicillin-resistant *S. aureus* (MRSA), extended spectrum beta-lactamase-producing Enterobacteriaceae (ESBLE-E), and carbapenem-resistant Enterobacteriaceae (CRE). VRE infection and colonization are increasing problems in liver patients and are associated with higher morbidity and mortality. Although there is no effective agent for VRE decolonization unlike MRSA, isolation and effective infection control measures, do help to control the spread. Eradication of MRSA colonization with nasal mupirocin ointment and chlorhexidine washes must be used to avoid infection. In the last decades, CRE is an emerging new superbug that is posing a serious threat to immunocompromised hosts. In endemic areas, CRE colonization and infection, particularly those due to carbapenem-resistant *Klebsiella pneumoniae* (CRKP), have become increasingly common in patients with liver

Table 10.1 **Pre-Transplant Infectious Disease Routine Screening Test for Liver Transplant Candidates and for Potential Donors**

	SCREENING TEST FOR TRANSPLANT CANDIDATE AND DONOR
*Screening for colonization of MDRO	Rectal swabs or stool culture: (CPE, VRE) Nasal, axilla, groin swab culture: MRSA
*Tuberculosis	*Mycobacterium tuberculosis*: Tuberculin and IGRA test
Syphilis	Rapid plasma reagin (RPR) or other serological test for syphilis
CMV	CMV IgG antibody
EBV	EBV IgG antibody
HIV	HIV 1 & 2 antibody & HIV antigen combo
HTLV I &II	HTLV I & II antibody
HBV	HBV surface antigen (HBSAG)
	HBV total core antibody (HBCAB) & HBSAB
HCV	Hepatitis C virus antibody (Anti-HCV IgG)
HEV	HEV RNA, HEV antibody
Parasitic infections	Toxoplasma IgG antibody Strongyloides serology in endemic areas
*Endemic mycoses	Coccidioidomycosis serology in endemic areas

* Screening should be considered in transplant candidates.
Abbreviations: MDRO: multidrug-resistant organism, VRE: vancomycin-resistant *Enterococcus faecium*, MRSA: methicillin-resistant *S. aureus*, CPE: carbapenemase-producing Enterobacteriaceae, IGRA: interferon gamma release assay, CMV: Cytomegalovirus, EBV: Epstein-Barr virus, HPV: human papilloma virus, HIV: human immunodeficiency virus, HBV: hepatitis B virus, HCV: hepatitis C virus.

disease and transplant recipients. Our experience shows that pre-transplant screening of CRE have significant impact on reducing the spread and infection rate of CRE in LT candidates and recipients. CRE colonization of donors or recipients is not a contraindication for transplant, while knowing the status of CRE colonization allows the appropriate management and prompt isolation and treatment of recipients in order to avoid transmission or infection.

- **Latent syphilis:** Potential LT candidates are screened for latent syphilis with a rapid plasma reagin (RPR) assay. If the results are positive, the patient should undergo a specific treponemal test (fluorescent treponemal antibody absorption test or micro hemagglutination assay for Treponema pallidum).

Positive RPR assay result with positive treponemal test results should be considered an indication of active or latent syphilis and should be treated according to standard guidelines.

• **Latent mycobacterial infection:** The patient's city and country of origin, as well as all prior sites of residence, is useful to assess the likelihood of asymptomatic exposure to *Mycobacterium tuberculosis*, parasites, and endemic fungi. A history of the child's contact with tuberculosis within or outside the family, animal exposure and hobbies may reveal other infection risks [5]. Transplant candidates who have resided in areas where tuberculosis is endemic should be evaluated using available assays and radiologic screening. Latent infection with *Mycobacterium tuberculosis* can be detected by skin testing with purified protein derivative (PPD), or by screening tests using interferon-gamma release assays (Quantiferon®-TB Gold test or ELISPOT). Both tests have been validated for screening in human immunodeficiency virus (HIV) infected patients but the efficacy of such testing in patients who may be immunocompromised as a result of pre-transplant organ dysfunction, is not well studied. Patients with positive PPD test and IGRA results should be considered for prophylactic therapy with isoniazid (INH) under expert supervision due to risk of hepatotoxicity. If transplantation is urgent, a patient may be listed prior to completion of prophylactic treatment but should continue INH therapy after transplantation with careful monitoring of liver function tests and cyclosporine or tacrolimus levels.

LATENT VIRAL INFECTION

Although a number of viral infections have been transmitted through donor organ transplantation, routinely tested viruses for both LT candidates and donors are CMV, EBV, HIV, VZV, HBV, and HCV. However, there is considerable center-to-center variation for screening of other viruses, for example, herpes simplex virus (HSV), human T-lymphotropic virus (HTLV I/II), HEV, and human herpes viruses 6, 7, and 8 (HHV6, 7, 8).

10.4 PRE-TRANSPLANT VACCINATION

Transplant candidates and recipients are at increased risk of vaccine-preventable infections because of immunosuppression. However, it is not uncommon for children requiring transplantation to have received inadequate or no immunizations pre-transplantation. Verifying immunization status and updating vaccinations are important steps in the pre-transplant evaluation. Every effort should be made to immunize children before transplant, early in the course of their disease before placing them on the waiting list for transplantation. The immune response is better before transplantation compared to after transplantation. Following transplantation children are on immunosuppressive medications, which further decreases antibody titres compared to control populations. All the available vaccines should be administered according to normal immunization schedules and other vaccines recommended for LT candidates (Table 10.2).

Live vaccines can safely be given ≥4 weeks and inactivated vaccines ≥2 weeks before the transplant. Ideally if patient listed for transplant and is given live

Table 10.2 **Vaccines for Children before and after Liver Transplantation**

VACCINE	LA/OR I VACCINES	COMMENTS
DPT (diphtheria pertussis and tetanus)	I	Minimum age is 2 months. Primary course of three doses at 1 month interval, and two boosters.
IPV (inactivated polio vaccine)	I	
Hib (*Haemophilus influenzae* type b)	I	Three doses at monthly interval for less than one year. One dose recommended if given after 2 years of age.
Rotavirus (RV)	LA	Two doses of RV vaccine (Rotarix) at 1-month interval for all infants. The maximum age for this vaccine is 6 months.
Pneumococcal conjugate vaccine (PCV) 13 serotypes	I	Three doses before 1 year. In unimmunized children after 1 year, two doses are recommended. When children are behind on PCV13 schedule, minimum interval for doses given to children >2 years is 2 months.
Pneumococcal polysaccharide vaccine (PPV23)	I	Immunogenic in children after 2 years of age. Should give PPV 8 weeks after PCV13 and to repeat dose after 5 years.
Meningococcal B	I	Minimum age is 2 months. Two doses at a 2-month interval. One dose is recommended if given after 1 year of age.

(Continued)

Table 10.2 **Vaccines for Children before and after Liver Transplantation (Continued)**

VACCINE	LA/OR I VACCINES	COMMENTS
Meningococcal C	I	Minimum age is 3 months. One dose is recommended if given after 1 year of age.
Meningococcal ACWY	I	Recommended age 10–18 years.
Inactivated influenza	I	Annual immunization before start of influenza seasons.
Hepatitis A	I	Minimum age 1 year, two doses at 6-month intervals. Immunoglobulin prophylaxis is indicated for, non-responders to active immunization in case of high risk of exposure (e.g., travel to endemic areas, infection of contacts).
Hepatitis B	I	Minimum age is 2 month, three doses at monthly interval. Antibody measurement should be done 1 month after the final dose. Do the antibody level before and after transplant.
*Measles, mumps and rubella (MMR)	LA	Normal age at 1 year, but if child listed for transplant at age of ≤1 year, can give vaccine after 6 months of age. One should consider doing measles IgG levels to rule out presence of maternal antibodies, which can interfere with immune response to vaccine. Complete immunization at least 4 weeks before LTX.
*Varicella zoster virus	LA	
Human papillomavirus vaccine (HPV)	I	Minimum age 12 years, two doses 6–24 months apart.

* All post-liver transplant recipients can have killed vaccines according to recommended immunization guide for immunocompromised patients. If unable to get vaccine at recommended ages, should follow catch-up immunization schedule.
Abbreviations: Live attenuated (LA), Inactivated (I), Liver transplantation (LTX).

vaccines, the child should be suspended from the transplant list for at least 4 weeks. The aim should be to complete immunizations at least 4 weeks before transplantation. MMR and varicella immunizations can be given from the age of 6 months onwards if the patient is listed for transplant before the age of one year. Two doses of MMR and varicella are recommended one month apart if recipient is antibody naïve for these viruses. It is also imperative to determine if the donor has received live vaccinations during the past 4 weeks against: varicella, MMR, BCG, cholera (oral vaccine), yellow fever, and Salmonella typhi (oral vaccine) or polio (oral vaccine) and influenza (inhaled live vaccine).

10.5 POST-TRANSPLANT VACCINATION

In general, all the killed vaccines can be resumed after transplant. However these may not be sufficiently immunogenic because of the effect of immunosuppressive therapy. Although there is no consensus as to the ideal time to vaccinate after transplantation, most centers restart vaccinations at approximately 6 months after transplantation in patients who are on standard immunosuppressive regimens. Historically, live attenuated vaccines (measles, mumps, rubella, and varicella) have not been recommended after transplant because of concern of vaccine strain induced illness in an immunocompromised patient. However recent studies have demonstrated safety and immunogenicity of live vaccines in select PLTR. Many transplant centers will do routine pre-transplant serology for vaccine-preventable diseases such as Hepatitis B, Varicella, measles, mumps and rubella to guide individual vaccine recommendations. Also with increasing outbreak of measles and decreasing herd immunity secondary to vaccine refusal, it is important to reassess if live vaccines should be contraindicated after transplant. The small theoretical risk of acquiring infection from live vaccines may be outweighed by risk of community exposure for pediatric. It is also important to immunise the child's immediate household contacts and healthcare workers.

10.6 INTRA- OR PERIOPERATIVE ANTIMICROBIAL PROPHYLAXIS IN PLTR

Preoperative antibiotics are administered prior to performing surgery to help decrease the risk of postoperative infections. The timing of antibiotic administration may vary, but the goal of administering preoperative systemic prophylactic antibiotics is to have the concentration in the tissues at its highest at the start and during surgery. The appropriate choice of antibiotic selection includes antibiotics which cover most organisms we want to target and have narrow spectrum of activity. Further the antibiotics choice is also based on multiple other factors including cost, safety, and ease of administration, pharmacokinetic profile, bactericidal activity, and hospital resistance patterns, and epidemiology of organisms. By addressing all of these factors during antibiotic selection, surgical site infections (SSIS) and postoperative infections are minimized. There is no universal consensus on type of antibiotic and appropriate duration of surgical antibiotic prophylaxis in LTX. Currently, there is no data to support the recommendations of a universal antibiotic prophylaxis protocol rather than an antibiotic regimen is individualized to a patient's comorbidities. In a European international multicentre survey on the current practice of perioperative antibiotic prophylaxis of 20 European PLTX centers, demonstrated great heterogeneity regarding all aspects of postoperative antimicrobial treatment, surveillance, and prevention of infections. The broad-spectrum regimens were the standard in 10 (50%) of centers and less frequent in the 16 (80%) centers with an infectious disease specialist. The duration ranged mainly between 24–48 h and 3–5 days in the absence and 3–5 days or 6–10 days in the presence of risk factors. Strategies regarding antifungal, antiviral, adjunctive antimicrobial, and surveillance strategies varied widely.

10.7 INFECTIONS AFTER LIVER TRANSPLANTATION IN CHILDREN

The incidence of infectious complications after LTX varies widely, but studies have reported infection rates ranging from 40% to 80% within the first year post-transplant. Bacterial infections account for most post-transplant infections (up to 70%), followed by viral and fungal infections. Liver transplant recipients (LTR) of deceased donor has higher rate of infections in comparison to living donor. The timing and risk of infections in LTR are determined by the intensity of exposure to infectious agents in a hospital or the community and level of immunosuppression. The net state of immunosuppression depends on the dose, duration and choice of immunosuppressive medications, underlying immune deficiencies and other risk factors. The timing of specific infections after LT historically has been divided in three time frames (Table 10.3).

10.8 COMMONLY ENCOUNTERED INFECTIONS AFTER LIVER TRANSPLANTATION AND MANAGEMENT

10.8.1 INFECTIONS IN FIRST MONTH AFTER LIVER TRANSPLANTATION

In the first month after LTX, patient susceptibility to infection is affected by donor-derived infections, surgical complications, environment, immunosuppression, and antimicrobial prophylaxis (Table 10.3). Opportunistic infections

Table 10.3 **Timeline of Risk Factors and Infection Type after Liver Transplantation**

TIMELINE FOR VARIOUS INFECTIONS AFTER TRANSPLANT		
1ST MONTH	BETWEEN 1ST–6TH MONTH	AFTER 6TH MONTH
Bacterial infections: SSI, intra-abdominal abdomen (infected ascites, abscesses, cholangitis), BSI, urosepsis, respiratory tract, line related, MDRO – VRE, MRSA, CRE **Viral infection**: HSV, CMV **Fungal infection**: *Candida* spp., rarely *Aspergillus* spp. Donor-derived infections	**Opportunistic pathogens:** CMV, EBV, HSV, HHV6&7 Pneumocystis, *Nocardia* spp., *Aspergillus* spp. TB, *Toxoplasma gondii* and endemic mycoses, recurrent cholangitis	Community-acquired viral infections, RTI, UTI, recurrent cholangitis, opportunistic infections, varicella-zoster, late CMV disease, fungal infections, Aspergillus
RISK FACTORS FOR INFECTIONS AFTER TRANSPLANT		
Prolonged hospital stay before LT, underlying disease; ALF, autoimmune hepatitis, infected donor organ perfusion fluid, level and type of immunosuppression, PNF graft, HAT and biliary complications, prolonged ICU-stay, dialysis, prolonged ventilation, Roux-en-Y, re-transplantation, prior colonization with MDRO, indwelling vascular and urinary catheterization, donor-transmitted diseases, ECMO; extracorporeal circulation membrane oxygenation	*General risks*: Over-immunosuppression, D+/R- mismatch status for viruses, allograft rejection, repeated biliary tract manipulations, re-transplantation, prolonged hospitalization	*General risks*: Only high-risk patients include those with recurrent rejection and allograft dysfunction that would require intense immunosuppression

Abbreviations: SSI: surgical site infection, ALF: acute liver failure, BSI: blood stream infection, HAT: hepatic artery thrombosis, PNF: primary non-functioning graft, OPF: organ preservation fluid, MDRO: multidrug resistant organisms, CMV: cytomegalovirus, EBV: Epstein-Barr virus, HHV: human herpesvirus, HSV: herpes simplex virus, ECMO: extracorporeal circulation membrane oxygenation, RTI, respiratory tract infections; UTI, urinary tract infection.

are rare in this period unless the patient has been on immunosuppression before transplant, e.g., for autoimmune liver disease or re-transplant.

10.9 DONOR-DERIVED INFECTIONS

Unexpected donor-derived infections may be transmitted via contaminated organ perfusion fluid, or infected tissue or systemic infection of the donor. Mostly routinely tested donor-derived infections (CMV, EBV, HIV, HTLV1&2, HBV, HCV, HEV, and MDRO) testing relies on serology, NAT, and culture (Table 10.2). However, unexpected transmissions are more difficult to detect in deceased donor because of time limitations between organ procurement and transplantation, donor infectious disease work-up is not always complete. They often manifest within the first month after LTX. These can be of common infections (e.g., MRSA, multidrug-resistant Gram-negatives) or more unusual pathogens such as *Cryptococcus*, lymphocytic choriomeningitis virus, or microsporidium, or West Nile virus, dengue, arboviruses or ZIKA virus. Clinicians should investigate more thoroughly for rare pathogens for the patients with unusual clinical symptoms or persistent fever on antimicrobials and without a focus or source identified by routine clinical testing.

10.10 BACTERIAL INFECTIONS AFTER LTX

There remains a relatively high incidence of 40–80% of bacterial infections after PLTR. Bacterial infections are particularly common with Gram-negative organisms and enterococci being the most common Gram-positive organism. Prophylactic antibiotics should be targeted based on risk factors and epidemiology and rationalize duration based on post-transplant clinical course postoperatively. Signs of occult infection may range from an occult rise in inflammatory markers and liver enzymes to fulminant septic shock. If fever is present, suspect a collection of fluid as a focus of infection, line infection or rejection. Full septic screen including (blood and urine cultures), CMV, EBV DNA, fungal biomarker beta-d glucan (BDG), baseline blood counts, C-reactive protein and procalcitonin, and radiological investigations including chest X-ray and ultrasound should be done. Broad-spectrum antibiotics should be commenced immediately, whilst awaiting culture results. Antimicrobial stewardship allows de-escalation to narrow spectrum antibiotics for infections with sensitive organisms.

Most common sites of bacterial infections are; surgical site infections (SSI), intra-abdominal, biliary, pneumonia and urosepsis. Endogenous Gram-negative bacteria predominantly cause infections in the bowel or biliary system. Surgical complications like bile leak or hepatic artery thrombosis can first present as infection or sepsis, positive blood culture for gut-derived organisms and should prompt investigations to exclude these events.

10.11 MULTIDRUG RESISTANT ORGANISMS (MDRO) IN PLTR

Globally PLTR are potentially at higher risk for colonization and infection with MDRO due to the increased exposure to antibiotics and the hospital environment. Furthermore, these pathogens are often associated with outbreaks. The prevalence of MDRO colonization and infections varies from center to center. We have reported a relatively low prevalence of MDRO (33% colonization, 23% infection rate) in our cohort of patients in comparison to reported data of 40% from other pediatric and adult LTR studies. We showed a high colonization rate with MRSA and CRE at 10.4%, likely because of active surveillance pre- and post-LTX for colonization of these organisms. Although we had a high rate of colonization with MRSA and VRE, the infection rate was low particularly with VRE in comparison to pre-antimicrobial stewardship (AMS) era. Gram-negative MDRO proved to be more problematic and has been associated with a higher morbidity and mortality in children and adult patients before and after transplant. Among Gram-negative bacteria, non-Carbapenemase-producing (non-CP CRE) and Carbapenemase-producing Enterobacteriaceae (CPE) are a growing challenge not only in transplant patients, but represent a more global problem. The colonization rate due to CPE in our center was 6.2% during active surveillance, in comparison to 25% during the non-active surveillance period. Therapeutic options for treating CRE (especially for metallo beta-lactamase-producing coliforms) are limited and therefore prevention of CRE is crucial. In our experience, colonization with MDRO was an independent risk factor for infection after transplant similar to results observed in adult studies. We demonstrated that pre-transplant screening of CRE had a significant impact on reducing the spread and infection rate of CRE in LT candidates and recipients. In our center we treated most CRE infections successfully, using a combination therapy of high-dose meropenem for CRE with minimum inhibitory concentration of <16 μg/mL plus colistin or fosfomicin or rifampicin or linezolid.

The high burden of coliforms, *Pseudomonas*, and *Enterococcus* with rising antimicrobial resistance is worrisome and it is important to consider optimizing and individualizing antibiotics to all these patients. Most importantly with limited therapeutic options for MDRO in PLTR, focus should be directed toward the prevention of these infections and strict antimicrobial stewardship (AMS).

10.12 FUNGAL INFECTIONS

Invasive fungal infections (IFI) remain an important cause of morbidity and mortality in PLTR. There has been limited experience in managing these infections in the pediatric cohort. We previously reported that up to 40.5% of children within our cohort developed a fungal infection (FI) within 1 year of LTX. Management of IFI has improved in the last decade due to availability of new classes of drugs such as echinocandins, mould-active azoles, and use of fungal biomarkers (beta-d-glucan for many fungal infections and galactomannan antigen for aspergillosis) for early diagnosis. Systemic antifungals are used as prophylaxis, treatment of documented specific infections and for treatment of a suspected IFI, but in the absence of definite proof of IFI. The most common fungal infections in PLTR are due to *Candida* (90%), and *C. albicans* is the most common species. However, with increasing use of fluconazole for antifungal prophylaxis there is higher prevalence of non–*C. albicans* yeast such as *C. Glabrata, C. parapsilosis*, or *C. krusei*. Risk factors for *Candida* include prolonged or repeat operation, re-transplantation, high intraoperative transfusion requirements, renal failure, prolonged broad spectrum antibiotic exposure, bowel perforation or biliary complications, CMV infection, choledochojejunostomy, and *Candida* colonization. Antifungal prophylaxis in LTR at high risk of developing IFI is widely agreed on, but there is no universal consensus on the type of antifungal agent and duration. Fluconazole and echinocandins are recommended for prophylaxis, but increasingly associated with resistance.

Invasive Aspergillus (IA) is the second most common cause of IFI in LTR. Compared with candidiasis, aspergillosis usually occurs later in the post-transplant period. Associated mortality varies from 30–100% in LTR. Risk factors for IA are severe prolonged neutropenia, bone marrow failure, fulminant hepatic failure, CMV infection, chronic lung disease with colonization of *Aspergillus*, building works in the close vicinity of transplant ward and ECMO. The LTR with risk factors for IA should be considered for mould active antifungal prophylaxis either posaconazole/voriconazole or caspofungin. Voriconazole remains the drug of choice to treat IA; isavuconazole and liposomal amphotericin B are alternative antifungals. Among all azoles voriconazole is the most hepatotoxic and interacts with calcineurin inhibitors. Its use can cause increase in tacrolimus concentration that require dosage adjustment. This drug-drug interaction can be attributed to a strong inhibitory effect on cytochrome P450–3A4 activity by voriconazole. When voriconazole and tacrolimus are co-administered, close monitoring of tacrolimus blood levels is recommended. Role of combination antifungals for primary treatment remains controversial. However in our experience initial combination antifungal therapy proved useful and effective for proven IFI. We used combination therapy until there is improvement clinically, and on imaging followed by long-term oral antifungal till full resolution. Risk factors for invasive candidiasis (IC) and IA continue to evolve, and thus strategies for their prevention should be constantly updated and targeted.

The early diagnosis of IFI is crucial for effective treatment. The diagnosis of IFI is challenging because current diagnostic methods lack sensitivity and specificity. The standard diagnostic methods include direct microscopic examination of clinical samples, culture, histopathology and imaging. However non-culture methods such as biomarkers beta-d-glucan (BDG) or galactomannan

(GM), or molecular tests are increasingly used as an adjunct for the diagnosis of IFI. BDG is a major component of fungal cell wall is useful in diagnosis for invasive candidiasis, IA, *Pneumocystis jiroveci* and other many fungal infections thus not specific. The GM assay is specific and sensitive test for diagnosis of IA, although it is also found in cell walls of *Histoplasma capsulatum* and *Fusarium* spp. In select cases of abnormal lesions in the lung on imaging, obtaining secretions and biopsies via bronchoscopic approach may be helpful for diagnosis of IA. Although GM can be tested in serum, CSF or pleural fluid but testing in bronchoalveolar lavage (BAL) is highly specific for diagnosis of IA. In PLTR few studies have shown the limited accuracy of BDG and GM in diagnosis of IFI and there is need for further evaluation of these tests in high-risk transplant recipients. Serological testing for fungal antibodies has more value in diagnosis of endemic mycoses. Early biopsy or aspiration should be considered in suspected tissue invasive fungal infection (brain, liver, spleen, oesophagus and skin). Beside microscopy and culture, it is crucial to do histology, fungal stain and PCR.

10.13 COMMON VIRAL INFECTIONS AFTER LIVER TRANSPLANTATION

10.13.1 CYTOMEGALOVIRUS (CMV) *INFECTION*

CMV is the most common infectious agent in the post-transplant period. The CMV serostatus of recipients and donors is the primary risk factor and antiviral prophylaxis is recommended for high-risk patients. The risk of infection is stratified by recipient and donor serostatus as seropositive donors with seronegative recipients (D^+/R^-), seropositive donors with seropositive recipients (D^+/R^+), seronegative donors with seropositive recipients (D^-/R^+), and seronegative donors with seronegative recipients (D^-/R^-). The PLTR with D^+/R^- serostatus are at the highest risk of CMV infection and disease, and should receive antiviral prophylaxis. Also, D^-/R^+ is a moderate risk because seronegative grafts when exposed to seropositive recipients are at risk of developing rejection or high rate of hepatitis. An alternative strategy that can be employed is one of close surveillance for infection and reactivation. Children with past CMV infections continue to have an increased risk of reactivation, in addition to the risk of acquiring a disease from a different strain of CMV if the donor is also positive. The CMV viral load should be routinely performed upon clinical suspicion. However, tissue-invasive CMV disease is not associated with CMV viraemia and requires confirmation by tissue pathology. Intravenous ganciclovir or oral valganciclovir are equivalent treatments, and the duration of treatment depends on factors including CMV viral load, tissue pathology, and clinical response. Patients should be monitored throughout therapy for renal dysfunction and bone marrow suppression. Patients should continue to have weekly CMV levels – if CMV viremia confirmed, increase frequency to treatment dose (BD) and treat until two CMV levels are reported negative.

10.14 EBV INFECTION AND POST-TRANSPLANT LYMPHOPROLIFERATIVE DISEASE

A majority (60–80%) of PLTR are EBV seronegative at transplantation, and more than 75% of them develop a primary infection in the first 6 months after transplantation. In the case of EBV-seropositive recipients, only 20–30% of them become reinfected. EBV infection can range from mononucleosis to frank non-Hodgkin lymphoma. The most serious complication after transplant is post-transplant lymphoproliferative disease (PTLD) and mainly occur in PLTR. The primary EBV infection, D+R- serostatus for EBV, immunosuppression and certain underlying autoimmune disorders were found to increase the risk for PTLD. The most effective intervention in case of high EBV DNA is reduction or cessation of immunosuppression but can increase the risk of graft loss. More recently, the anti-CD20 monoclonal antibody (rituximab) has been shown to improve survival in various transplant populations with B-cell PTLD. WHO pathology classification of a tissue biopsy remains the gold standard for PTLD diagnosis; optimal staging procedures are uncertain. Other therapeutic options are chemotherapy, surgery or radiotherapy. EBV-directed cytotoxic T cells have shown promise in the management of PTLD but its clinical use is limited by lack of technical facilities. EBV-DNA monitoring has played an important role in the diagnosis and management of EBV–associated PTLD and should be done in all high-risk patients in the first-year post-LTX.

10.15 COMMON INFECTIONS 6 MONTHS POST-LIVER TRANSPLANTATION

Late in the post-transplant period, most PLTR are on lower immunosuppression reducing the risk of infections. The community acquired infections, e.g., viruses and food borne gastroenteritis are most common. Occasionally, some recipients will develop primary or late CMV infection, papillomavirus and relapsing viral infections. Subgroup of PLTR who are on higher level of maintenance immunosuppression or have biliary/arterial complications suffer from recurrent infections requiring repeated hospitalizations and antimicrobial therapy. They are at risk of developing colonization and infection by MDRO and other common opportunistic pathogens (e.g., *P. jiroveci*, *Aspergillus* species). Recurrent cholangitis is one of the late infectious complications in fewer numbers of PLTR particularly those who develop biliary complications. Community-acquired pneumonia (CAP) occurs in a significant proportion of patients late after LTX. The main agents causing CAP are viruses (influenza, RSV, rhinoviruses) and bacterial pathogens are less common (*Streptococcus pneumoniae*, *Haemophilus influenza*, and the atypical pathogens such as *Mycoplasma pneumoniae* and *Chlamydia pneumoniae*). Other late infectious complications most commonly reported are late CMV and herpes zoster. Rarely infections due *Cryptosporidium*, molds (mucormycosis), and common diseases (herpes zoster, HSV) or TB of unusual severity are also reported.

10.16 INFECTION PREVENTION STRATEGIES IN THE POST-TRANSPLANT PERIOD

The patient and their close contacts should be instructed to have strict hand hygiene, environmental cleanliness, and contact precaution with ill persons, especially during the early postoperative period of maximal immunosuppression. Close contacts of recipients should keep their immunizations up to date in an effort to establish herd immunity and thus decrease the possibility of infection in the PLTR. Passive immunity and treatment should be considered for PLTR following contact with varicella zoster virus, herpes simplex virus (HSV), and measles.

10.17 VARICELLA ZOSTER VIRUS CONTACT

Chickenpox contact is a common issue for PLTR. Exposure is defined as contact with a case 48 hours or less before the onset of the rash up until the time that the lesions are crusted over. Relevant contacts are those within the household, in the same classroom, or any face-to-face contact for ≥15 mins. PLTR with history of chickenpox contact should have varicella antibody titre done as soon as possible, if there is no recent serology available within 3 days of exposure. If Varicella antibody is positive, no action is required; if negative, and within 7 days of contact consider varicella immunoglobulin and oral aciclovir prophylaxis.

10.18 HERPES SIMPLEX VIRUS CONTACT

For contact with household person with active cold sore, healthcare professionals should consider oral aciclovir prophylaxis for children.

10.19 MEASLES CONTACT

Normal human immunoglobulin should be given to non-immune child who is in contact with measles ideally within 6 days of contact. The infectious period is from the beginning of the prodromal period to 4 days after the appearance of the rash.

Risks related to the parent's occupation, hobbies, social and travel habits, and animal contacts should also be explored. The key infection-prevention strategies in LTR involved improving primary or pre-emptive prophylaxis with antimicrobials and vaccination, adherence to infection-control recommendations in healthcare or home settings, promoting healthy behaviour and risk reduction in various settings after transplant, e.g., pretravel consultation. Travel history may provide insight into exposure to contaminated food and water (listeria, cryptosporidium), soil (*Aspergillus* or *Nocardia*), birds (*Cryptococcus*), and geographically restricted mycoses (*Blastomyces dermatitidis, Coccidioides immitis, Paracoccidioides* species, and *Histoplasma capsulatum*), in addition to outbreaks of respiratory viruses and arthropod-borne diseases.

10.20 CONCLUSIONS

Comprehensive pre-transplant infectious disease work-up, immunizations, and perioperative and prophylactic antimicrobials are vital to decreasing the rate of infections after liver transplantation. Screening of recipients and donors is crucial to minimise the reactivation or the risk of transmission. In the post-transplant period, diagnostic work-up and therapy (empirical or targeted) should be performed by an expert with experience in transplant infectious diseases within a multidisciplinary team. Early diagnosis and treatment of infections are usually associated with improved outcomes.

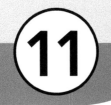

11 Future developments

Future developments in pediatric transplantation hold the promise of further improving outcomes, increasing organ availability, and enhancing the overall care of pediatric patients with end-stage disease. Some of the potential advancements and areas of focus in this field include:

1. *Minimally invasive techniques*: There is ongoing research to refine and expand the use of minimally invasive surgical techniques for pediatric transplantation. Minimally invasive approaches can lead to reduced surgical trauma, quicker recovery times, and improved cosmetic outcomes, making them particularly advantageous for pediatric patients.

2. *Living donor transplantation (LDT)*: As the demand for pediatric transplants continues to exceed the supply of deceased donor organs, living donor transplantation is likely to play a more significant role in the future. Efforts are being made to enhance the safety of living donors and expand the pool of potential donors, including the use of extended criteria donors and partial grafts in liver transplantation, from living donors.

3. *Regenerative medicine*: The field of regenerative medicine holds great potential for transplantation. Researchers are exploring the use of stem cells and tissue engineering to create bioengineered organs or grafts. This could revolutionize the transplantation process by reducing the need for donor organs and potentially eliminating the need for immunosuppressive medications.

4. *Artificial devices*: Development and refinement of artificial support systems are underway. These devices aim to bridge the gap between liver failure and transplantation by providing temporary liver support, allowing time for the liver to recover or for a suitable donor organ to become available.

5. *Immune tolerance induction*: Advancements in immune tolerance induction techniques may enable transplant recipients to better tolerate the transplanted organs without the need for long-term immunosuppressive medications. This can reduce the risk of complications associated with immunosuppression and improve the long-term health of transplant recipients.

DOI: 10.1201/9781003341741-11

6. *Personalized medicine*: The use of genetic profiling and personalized medicine approaches may help tailor transplant strategies to individual patients, optimizing organ allocation and minimizing the risk of rejection.

7. *Donor organ preservation*: Improvements in organ preservation techniques, such as machine perfusion, may increase the viability of donor organs, allowing for longer transport times and potentially expanding the donor pool.

8. *Post-transplant management*: There is a growing focus on long-term post-transplant care, including the management of complications and optimizing the health and well-being of pediatric transplant recipients throughout their lives.

Overall, the future of pediatric transplantation is bright, with ongoing research and innovations aimed at improving outcomes, expanding donor options, and providing the best possible care for children with end-stage disease. Collaboration among researchers, clinicians, and healthcare providers will be key to driving these developments and ensuring that pediatric liver transplant recipients continue to have a higher quality of life and improved long-term survival.

12 Summary

Pediatric abdominal organ transplantation is a worldwide strategy which should be expanded to centers that are willing to move forward with transplantation. Centers should explore the kidney transplantation pathway, moving forward into complex kidney transplantation; subsequently proceeding with liver transplantation at the same time of complex hepatobiliary surgery, challenging kidney transplants and pancreatic or simultaneous kidney pancreas transplant, although the latter is uncommon in the pediatric population. Finally, small bowel transplant should be an alternative considered on patients who meet the criteria, and it is important to mention that multivisceral or isolated bowel or combined bowel transplant should be performed in patients, not a lifesaving procedure, but as a quality-of-life transplant procedure.

We have discussed the different types of abdominal solid organs used for transplant, albeit the list of transplants and alternatives can be as wide as the problem is. We consider that transplant boundaries are continuously being surpassed and patients should always receive the possibility for transplantation only in case there is no contraindication.

It has been demonstrated that a good alternative for organ transplant to reduce the waiting list is living donation.

We strongly suggest trying to proceed with organ transplantation preemptively in organ failure in order to provide better outcomes for children.

DOI: 10.1201/9781003341741-12

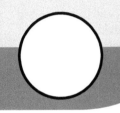

Bibliography

1. Chinnakotla S, et al. Total pancreatectomy and islet auto-transplantation in children for chronic pancreatitis: Indication, surgical techniques, post-operative management and long-term outcomes. Ann Surg. 2014;260(1):56–64.
2. Gentry SE, Montgomery RA, Segev DL. Kidney paired donation: Fundamentals, limitations and expansions. Am J Kidney Dis. 2011;57(1):144–151.
3. Busuttil RW, et al. *Transplantation of the liver*, 3rd edition. Philadelphia: Saunders, Imprint of Elsevier, 2015. ISBN: 978-1-4557-0268-8.
4. Ishak KG. Hepatocellular carcinoma associated with inherited metabolic diseases. Eti Path Treat Hepatocell Carcin N Am. 1991:91–103.
5. Manzia TM, et al. Glycogen storage disease type IA and VI associated with hepatocellular carcinoma: Two case reports. Transplant Proc. 2011;43(4):1181–1183.
6. Reyes JD, et al. Liver transplantation and chemotherapy for hepatoblastoma and hepatocellular cancer in childhood and adolescence. J Pediatr. 2000;136(6):795–804.
7. Browne M, et al. Survival after liver transplantation for hepatoblastoma: A 2-center experience. J Pediatr Surg. 2008;43(11):1973–1981.
8. Rela M, et al. Auxiliary partial orthotopic liver transplantation for Crigler-Najjar syndrome type I. Ann Surg. 1999;229(4):565–569.
9. Fox IJ, et al. Treatment of the Crigler-Najjar syndrome type I with hepatocyte transplantation. N Eng J Med. 1998;338(20):1422–1426.
10. Van der Veere CN, et al. Current therapy for Crigler-Najjar syndrome type 1: Report of a world registry. Hepatol. 1996;24(2):311–315.
11. Whitington PF, Alonso AE. *Fulminant hepatitis and acute liver failure*. Oxford: Oxford University Press, 2003, pp. 107–126.
12. Alonso E, Squires R, Whitington P. Acute liver failure in children. In: Suchy F, Sokol R, Balistreri W, editors. *Liver disease in children*. Cambridge: Cambridge University Press, 2007, pp. 71–96. doi:10.1017/CBO9780511547409.007.
13. Squires Jr RH, et al. Acute liver failure in children: The first 348 patients in the pedlatric acute liver failure study group. J Pediatr. 2006;148(5):652–658.
14. Noble-Jamieson G, et al. Liver transplantation for hepatic cirrhosis in cystic fibrosis. J R Soc Med. 1996;89:31–37.
15. Mack DR, et al. Clinical denouement and mutation analysis of patients with cystic fibrosis undergoing liver transplantation for biliary cirrhosis. J Pediatr. 1995;127(6):881–887.
16. Colombo C, et al. Liver disease in cystic fibrosis. J Pediatr Gastroenterol Nutr. 2006;S49–S55.
17. Barr ML, et al. A report of the Vancouver forum on the care of the live organ donor: Lung, liver, pancreas, and intestine data and medical guidelines. Transplantation. 2006;81(10):1373–1385.

18. Nakamuta M, et al. Short-term intensive treatment for donors with hepatic steatosis in living-donor liver transplantation. Transplantation. 2005;80(5):608–612.
19. Liu C, et al. Increasing donor body weight to prevent small-for-size syndrome in living donor liver transplantation. World J Surg. 2010;34(10):2401–2408.
20. Van Belle T, Coppieters K, Von Herrath M. Type 1 diabetes: Etiology, immunology, and therapeutic strategies. Physiol Rev. 2011;91:79–118.
21. Nathan DM. Long-term complications of diabetes mellitus. N Eng J Med. 1993;385:1676–1685.
22. (DCCT): 3DCCT Research Group Diabetes Control and Complications Trial. The effect of intensive diabetes treatment in long-term complications in IDDM. N Eng J Med. 1993;329:977–986.
23. McDonald SP, Craig JC. Long-term survival of children with end-stage renal disease. N Eng J Med. 2004;350:2654–2662.
24. Nissel R, Brazda I, Feneberg R. Effect of renal transplantation in childhood on longitudinal growth and adult height. Kidney Int. 2004;66:792–800.
25. Riano-Galan I, Malaga S, Rajmil L. Quality of life of adolescents with end-stage renal disease and kidney transplant. Pediatr Nephrol. 2009;24:1561–1568.
26. Motoyama O, Kawamura T, Aikawa A. Head circumference and development in young children after renal transplantation. Pediatr Int. 2009;51:71–74.
27. Nagarathnam M, Sivakumar V, Latheef SAA. Burden, coping mechanisms, and quality of life among caregivers of hemodialysis and peritoneal dialysis undergoing and renal transplant patients. Indian J Psychiatry. 2019;61(4):380–388.
28. National Kidney Foundation. K/DOQI clinical practice guidelines for chronic kidney disease: Evaluation, classification, and stratification. Am J Kidney Dis. 2002;39:S1.
29. Wong C, Warady BA. *Chronic kidney disease in children: Definition, epidemiology, etiology, and course*, 2019. https://www.ncbi.nlm.nih.gov/pmc/articles/PMC4957724/.
30. NAPRTCS. *2008 Annual report*. Rockville, MD: EMMES, 2008.
31. Ardissino G, Dacco V, Testa S. Epidemiology of chronic renal failure in children: Data from the ItalKid project. Pediatrics. 2003;11:382.
32. Wong CJ, Moxey-Mims M, Jerry-Fluker J. CKiD (CKD in children) prospective cohort study: A review of current findings. Am J Kidney Dis. 2012;60:1002.
33. Mong H, Ismaili K, Collart F. Clinical characteristics and outcomes of children with stage 3–5 chronic kidney disease. Pediatr Nephrol. 2010;25:935.
34. Morris PJ, Knechtle SJ. *Kidney transplantation*, 7th edition. Philadelphia: Elsevier Saunders, 2014.
35. U.S Renal Data System. *2011 Annual data report: Atlas of chronic kidney disease and end-stage renal disease in the United States*. Bethesda, MD: USRDS, National Institutes of Health, National Insittues of Diabetes and Digestive Kidney Diseases, 2011.
36. Furth SL, Abraham AG, Jerry-Fluker J. Metabolic abnormalities, cardiovascular disease risk factors, and GFR decline in children with chronic kidney disease. USRDS. Clin J Am Soc Nephrol. 2011;6:2132.
37. Crump C, et al. Preterm birth and risk of chronic kidney disease from childhood into mid-adulthood: National cohort study. BMJ. 2019;365:1346.
38. Ardissino G, Testa S, Dacco V. Puberty is associated with increased deterioration of renal function in patients with CKD: Data from the ItalKid project. Arch Dis Child. 2012;97:885.
39. Warady BA, Abraham AG, Schwartz, GJ. Predictors of rapid progression of glomerular and nonglomerular kidney disease in children and adolescents: The chronic kidney disease in children (CKiD) cohort. Am J Kidney Dis. 2015;65:878.

40. Querfeld U, Anarat A, Bayazit AK. The cardiovascular comorbidity in children with chronic kidney disease (4C) study: Objectives, design, and methodology. Clin J Am Soc Nephrol. 2010;5:1642.
41. Shroff R, Aitkenhead H, Costa N. Normal 25-hydroxyvitamin D levels are associated with less proteinuria and attenuate renal failure progression in children with CKD. J Am Soc Nephrol. 2016;27:314.
42. Staples AO, Greenbaum LA, Smith JM. Association between clinical risk factors and progression of chronic kidney disease in children. Clin J Am Soc Nephrol. 2010;5:2172.
43. Portale AA, Wolf MS, Messinger S. Fibroblast growth factor 23 and risk of CKD progression in children. Clin J Am Soc Nephrol. 2016;11:1989.
44. Rodenbach JE, Schneider MF, Furth SL. Hyperuricemia and progression of CKD in children and adolescents: The chronic kidney disease in children (CKiD) cohort study. Am J Kidney Dis. 2015;66:984.
45. ESCAPE Trial Group, Wuhl E, Trivelli A. Strict blood-pressure control and progression of renal failure in children. N Eng J Med. 2009;361:1639.
46. Rockville, MD, North American Pediatric Renal Transplant Cooperative Study (NAPRTCS): 2014 Annual Report. 2014. https://naprtcs.org/system/files/2014_Annual_Transplant_Report.pdf.
47. North American Pediatric Renal Trials and Collaborative Studies 2008 Annual Report. 2008. https://www.naprtcs.org/system/files/2008_Annual_CKD_Report.pdf.
48. Neu AM. Special issues in pediatric kidney transplantation. Adv Chronic Kidney Dis. 2006;13:62.
49. Cransberg K, Smits JM, Offner G. Kidney transplantation without prior dialysis in children: The Eurotransplant experience. Am J Transplant. 2006;6:1858.
50. McDonald R, Niaudet P, Kim MS. Kidney transplantation in children: General principles. *Up to Date*, 2019. https://www.uptodate.com.
51. Tyden G, Kumlien G, Berg UB. ABO-Incompatible kidney transplantation in children. Pediatr Transplant. 2011;15:502–504.
52. Stojanovic J, et al. Immune desensitization allow pediatric blood group incompatible kidney transplantation. Transplantation. 2017;101(6):1242–1246.
53. Sypek MP, et al. Optimizing outcomes in pediatric renal transplantation through the Australian paired kidney exchange program. Am J Transplant. 2017;17:534–541.
54. Summers DM, et al. Kidney donation after circulatory death (DCD): State of the art. Kidney Int. 2015;88:241–249.
55. Ibrahim M, et al. An international comparison of deceased donor kidney. Am J Transplant. 2020;20:1309–1322.
56. NHSBT. *Annual report on deceased donation and transplantation in paediatrics*. NHSBT, 2019. https://www.odt.nhs.uk/statistics-and-reports/paediatric-activity-reports/
57. Dale-Shall AW, Smith JM, McBride, MA. The relationship of donor source and age on short- and long-term allograft survival in pediatric renal transplantation. Pediatr Transplant. 2009;13:711.
58. Chandak P, et al. Insights in transplanting complex pediatric renal recipients with vascular anomalies. Transplantation, 2017;101(10):2562–2570.
59. Adamusiak A, et al. Desensitization protocol enabling pediatric crossmatch-positive renal transplantation: Successful HLa-antivody-incompatible renal transplantation of two highly sensitized children. Pediatr Nephrol. 2017;32:359–364.
60. Kucira LM, Sarathi H, Govindan P. Risk of window period HIV infection in high infectious risk donors: Systematic review and meta-analysis. Am J Transplant. 2011;11:1176–1187.

61. Kucirka LM, Sarathy H, Govindan P. Risk of window period hepatitis-C infection in high infectious risk donors: Systematic review and meta-analysis. Am J Transplant. 2011;11:1188–1200.
62. Kizilbash SJ, Rheault MN, Wang Q. Kidney transplant outcomes associated with the use of increased risk donors in children. Am J Transplant. 2019;13:1227–1234.
63. Damji S, Callaghan CJ, Loukopoulos I. Utilisation of small paediatric donor kidneys for transplantation. Pediatr Transplant. 2019;23:135–140.
64. Harmon WE, et al. The effect of donor age on graft survival in pediatric cadaver renal transplant recipients. Transplantation. 1992;54:232–237.
65. Van Heurn E, De Vries E. Kidney transplantation and donation in children. Pediatr Surg Int. 2009;25:385–393.
66. Metzger RA, Delmonico FL, Feng S. Expanded criteria donors for kidney transplantation. Am J Transplant. 2003;3(Suppl 4):114–125.
67. Sureshkumar KK, Reddy CS, Nghiem DD. Superiority of pediatric en bloc renal allografts over living donor kidneys: A long-term functional study. Transplantation. 2006;82:348–353.
68. Sharma A, Fisher RA, Cotterell AH. En bloc kidney transplantation from pediatric donors: comparable outcomes with living donor kidney transplantation. Transplantation. 2011;92:564–569.
69. Suneja M, et al. Small split pediatric kidneys to expand the donor pool: An analysis of scientific registry of transplant recipients data. Transplantation. 2019;103(12):2549–2557.
70. Cohen J, Rees A, Williams G. A prospective randomized controlled trial of perioperative antibiotic prophylaxis in renal transplantation. J Hosp Infect. 1988;11:357–363.
71. Evans CM, et al. Amoxycillin-clavulanic acid (Augmentin) antibiotic prophylaxis against wound infections in renal failure patients. J Antimicrob Chemother. 1988;22:363–369.
72. Darouiche RO, et al. Chlorhexidine-alcohol versus povidone-iodine for surgical-site antisepsis. N Engl J Med. 2010;362:18–26.
73. Hume DM. et al. Renal homotransplantation in man in modified recipients. Ann Surg. 1963;158:608–644.
74. Kuss R, Tsenturier J, Milliez P. Quelques essais de greffes du rein chez l'homme. Mem Acad Chir. 1951;77:755.
75. Starzl TE, et al. Technique of renal homotransplantation: Experience with 42 cases. Arch Surg. 1964;89:87–104.
76. West MS, et al. Renal pedicle torsion after simultaneous kidney-pancreas transplantation. J Am Coll Surg. 1998;187:80–87.
77. Montgomery JR, Berger JC, Warren, DS. Outcomes of ABO-incompatible kidney transplantation in the United States. Transplantation. 2012;93:603–609.
78. Tyden G, Kumlien G, Berg UB. ABO-Incompatible kidney transplantation in children. Pediatr Transplant. 2011;15:502–504.
79. Shimmura J, et al. Role of anti-A/B antibody titers in results of ABO-incompatible kidney transplantation. Transplantation. 2000;70:1331–1335.
80. Aikawa A, Hadano T, Ohara T. Donor specific antibody suppression in ABO incompatible kidney transplantation. Transplant Proc. 2001;33:395–397.
81. Park WD, Grande JP, Ninova D. Accommodation in ABO-incompatible kidney allografts, a novel mechanism of self-protection against antibody-mediated injury. Am J Transplant. 2003;3:952–960.

82. Chopek MW, Simmons RL, Platt JL. ABO-incompatible kidney transplantation: initial immunopathologic evaluation. Transplant Proc. 1987;19:4553–4557.
83. Van Hoek B, et al. Auxiliary versus orthotopic liver transplantation for acute liver failure. EURALT study group. European Auxiliary Liver Transplant Registry. J Hepatol. 1999;30:699–705.
84. Carrell A. Le technique opératoire des anastomoses vasculaires et la transplantation des viscères. Lyon Med. 1902;98:859–864.
85. Lee HM. Surgical techniques of renal transplantation. Kidney Transplant. 1979;145.
86. Lich R. Jr. Obstructive diseases of the urinary tract in children. J Ark Med Soc. 1961;58:127–130.
87. Pleass HC, et al. Urologic complications after renal transplantation: A prospective randomized trial comparing different techniques of ureteric anastomosis and the use of prophylactic ureteric stents. Transplant Proc. 1995;27:1091–1092.
88. Politano VA, Leadbetter WF. An operative technique for the correction of vesicoureteral reflux. J Urol. 1958;79:932–941.
89. Stevens A, Marshall V. Reimplantation of the ureter into the bladder. Surg Gynecol Obstet. 1943;77:585.
90. Benoit G, et al. Insertion of a double pigtail ureteral stent for the prevention of urological complications in renal transplantation: a prospective randomized study. J Urol. 1996;156:881–884.
91. Robert Kane MD, Harvey Solomon MD, Barry Friedman RN, et al. Studies of pediatric liver transplantation (SPLIT): Year 2000 outcomes. Transplantation. 2001;72(3):463–476.
92. Ng VL, et al. Outcomes of 5-year survivors of pediatric liver transplantation: Report on 461 children from a North American multicenter registry. Pediatrics. 2008;122:e1128–e1135.
93. Group SR. Immunosuppression: First transplant. SPLIT Annual Report. 2006: 1–11.
94. Ribes-Koninckx C, et al. Clinical outcome of hepatocyte transplantation in four pediatric patients with inherited metabolic diseases. Cell Transplant. 2012; 21(10):2267–2282.
95. Limbers CA, et al. Health-related quality of life in pediatric liver transplant recipients compared with other chronic disease groups. Pediatr Transplant. 2011;21(10):245–253.
96. Ng VL, et al. Health status of children alive 10 years after pediatric liver transplantation performed in the US and Canada: Report of the studies of pediatric liver transplantation experience. J Pediatr. 2012;160(5):820–826.
97. Miga D, et al. Survival after first esophageal variceal hemorrhage in patients with biliary atresia. J Pediatr. 2001;139(2):291–296.
98. Grosfeld JL, et al. The efficacy of hepatoportoenterostomy in biliary atresia. Surgery. 1989;106(4):692–700.
99. Lilly JR, et al. The surgery of biliary atresia. Ann Surg. 1989;210(3):289–294.
100. Emerick KM, Whitington PF. Partial external biliary diversion for intractable pruritus and xanthomas in Alagille syndrome. Hepatology. 2002;35(6):1501–1506.
101. Starzl TE, et al. Changing concepts: Liver replacement for hereditary tyrosinemia and hepatoma. J Pediatr. 1985;106(4):604–606.
102. Esquivel CO, et al. Liver transplantation for hereditary tyrosinemia in the presence of hepatocellular carcinoma. Transplant Proc. 1989;21:2445–2446.

103. Freese DK, et al. Early liver transplantation is indicated for tyrosinemia type I. Pediatr Gastroenterol Nutr. 1991;13(1):10–15.
104. Houlihan DD, et al. Review article: Liver transplantation for the pulmonary disorders of portal hypertension. Aliment Pharmacol Ther. 2013;37(2):183–194.
105. Porres-Aguilar M, et al. Portopulmonary hypertension and hepatopulmonary syndrome: A clinician-oriented overview. Eur Respir Rev. 2012;21(125):223–233.
106. Millan MT, et al. A 100% 2-year graft survival can be attained in high-risk 15-kg or smaller infant recipients of kidney allografts. Arch Surg. 2000; 135:1063–1068.
107. Irtan S, et al. Renal transplantation in children: Critical analysis of age related surgical complications. Pediatr Tranpslant. 2010;14:512–519.
108. Englesbe MJ, et al. Early urologic complications after pediatric renal transplant: A single-center experience. Transplantation. 2008;86:1560–1564.
109. Barrero R, et al. Vesicoureteral reflux after kidney transplantation in children. Pediatr Transplant. 2007;11:498–503.
110. Coran AG, et al. *Pediatric surgery*. Philadelphia: Elsevier, 2012. 978-0-323-07255-7.
111. Smith JM, et al. Contributions of the transplant registry: The 2006 annual report of the North American pediatric renal trials and collaborative studies (NAPRTCS). Pediatr Transplant. 2007;11:366–373.
112. Magee JC, et al. Pediatric transplantation in the United States, 1997–2006. Am J Transplant. 2008;8(4–2):935–945.
113. McDonald RA, Smith JM, Stablein D. Pretransplant peritoneal dialysis and graft thrombosis following pediatric kidney transplantation: A NAPRTCS report. Pediatr Transplant. 2003;7:204–208.
114. Benfield MR, et al. Changing trends in pediatric transplantation: 2001 annual report of the North American pediatric renal transplant cooperative study. Pediatr Transplant. 2003;7:321–335.
115. Magee JC, et al. Pediatric transplantation. Am J Transplant. 2004;4:54–71.
116. Sarwal MM, Cecka JM, Millan MT. Adult-size kidneys without acute tubular necrosis provide exceedingly superior long-term graft outcomes for infants and small children: A single center and UNOS analysis. United network for organ sharing. Transplantation. 2000;70:1728–1736.
117. Gaston RS, et al. Evidence for antibody-mediated injury as a major determinant of late kidney allograft failure. Transplantation. 2010;90:68–74.
118. Kelly WD, Lillehei RC, Merkel FK Allotransplantation of the pancreas and duodenum along with the kidney in diabetic nephropathy. Surgery. 1967;61:827–835.
119. Boggi U, Amorese G, Marchetti P. Surgical techniques for pancreas transplantation. Curr Opin Organ Transplant. 2010;15:102–111.
120. Boggi U, et al. A simplified technique for the en bloc procurement of abdominal organs that is suitable for pancreas and small-bowel transplantation. Surgery. 2004;135:629–641.
121. Marsh CK, et al. Combined hepatic and pancreaticoduodenal procurement for transplantation. Surg Gynecol Obstet. 1989;168:254–258.
122. Boggi U, et al. A new technique for retroperitoneal pancreas transplantation with portal-enteric drainage. Transplantation. 2005;79:1137–1142.
123. Boggi U, et al. Portal enteric-drained solitary pancreas transplantation without surveillance biopsy: Is it safe? Transplant Proc. 2004;36:1090–1092.
124. Benedetti E, et al. Successful living related simultaneous pancreas-kidney transplant between identical twins. Transplantation. 1999;67:915–918.

125. Guressner R, et al. Simultaneous pancreas-kidney transplantation from live donors. Ann Surg. 1997;226:471–482.
126. Sutherland DER, Goetz FC, Najarian JS. Pancreas transplants from living related donors. Transplantation. 1984;38:625–633.
127. Sutherland DER, Najarian J, Gruessner R. *Pancreas transplantation.* New York: McGraw-Hill, 2007, pp. 369–384.
128. Boggi U, et al. Segmental live donor pancreas transplantation: Review and critique of rationale, outcomes, and current recommendations. Clin Transplant. 2011;25:4–12.
129. Sutherland D. Extra-renal living donor transplants with special reference to segmental pancreas transplantation. Clin Transplant. 2011;25:1–3.
130. Drachenberg C., et al. Banff schema for grading pancreas allograft rejection: Working proposal by a multi-disciplinary international consensus panel. Am J Transplant. 2008;8:1237–1249.
131. Gaber L. Pancreas allograft biopsies in the management of pancreas transplant recipients: Histopathologic review and clinical correlations. Arch Pathol Lab Med. 2007;131:1192–1199.
132. Gruessner AC, Sutherland DER, Gruessner RWG. Pancreas transplantation in the United States: A review. Curr Opin Organ Transplant. 2010;15:93–101.
133. Douzdjian V, Ferrara D, Silvestri, G. Treatment strategies for insulin-dependent diabetics with ESRD: A cost-effectiveness decision analysis model. Am J Kidney Dis. 1998;31:794–802.
134. Fioretto P, et al. Reversal of lesions of diabetic nephropathy after pancreas transplantation. N Eng J Med. 1998;339:69–75.
135. Gross CR, Limwattananon C, Matthees BJ. Quality of life after pancreas transplantation: A review. Clin Transplant. 1998;12:351–361.
136. Navarro X, Sutherland DER, Kennedy WR. Long-term effects of pancreatic transplantation on diabetic neuropathy. Ann Neurol. 1997;42:727–736.
137. Stratta RJ. The economics of pancreas transplantation. Graft. 2000;3:19.
138. Tyden G, et al. Improved survival in patients with insulin-dependent diabetes mellitus and end-stage diabetic nephropathy 10 years after combined pancreas and kidney transplantation. Transplantation. 1999;67:645–648.
139. Zehrer CL, Gross CR. Quality of life of pancreas transplant recipients. Diabetologia. 1991;34:S145–S149.
140. Dendall DM, et al. Pancreas transplantation restores epinephrine response and symptom recognition during hypoglycemia in patients with long-standing type I diabetes and autonomic neuropathy. Diabetes. 2000;46:249–257.
141. Navarro X, et al. Neuropathy and mortality in diabetes: Influence of pancreas transplantation. Muscle Nerve. 1996;19:1009–1016.
142. Robertson RP, et al. Metabolic characterization of long-term successful pancreas transplants in type I diabetes. J Invest Med. 1996;44:549–555.
143. Troppmann C. Complications after pancreas transplantation. Curr Opin Organ Transplant. 2010;15:112–118.
144. Goulet O, Reummele F, Lacaille F. Irreversible intestinal failure. J Pediatr Gastroenterol Nutr. 2004;38:250–269.
145. Colomb V, et al. Long-term outcome of children receiving home parenteral nutrition: A 20-year single-center experience in 302 patients. J Pediatr Gastroenterol Nutr. 2007;44:347–353.
146. Tzakis AG, et al. 100 multivesicular transplants at a single center. Ann Surg. 2005;242:discussion 491–483.

147. Colomb V, et al. Central venous catheter-related infections in children on long-term home parenteral nutrition: Incidence and risk factors. Clin Nutr. 2000;19:355–359.

148. Beath S, et al. Collaborative strategies to reduce mortality and morbidity in patients with chronic intestinal failure including those who are referred for small bowel transplantation. Transplantation. 2008;85:1378–1384.

149. Grant D, et al. 2003 report of the intestine transplant registry: A new era has dawned. Ann Surg. 2005;241:607–613.

150. Colomb V, et al. Role of lipid emulsions in cholestasis associated with long-term parenteral nutrition in children. J Parenter Enteral Nutr'. 2000;24:345–350.

151. Goulet O, et al. A new intravenous fat emulsion containing soybean oil, medium-chain triglycerides, olive oil, and fish oil: A single-center, double-blind randomized study on efficacy and safety in pediatric patients receiving home parenteral nutrition. J Parenter Enteral Nutr. 2010;34:485–495.

152. Gura KM, et al. Reversal of parenteral nutrition-associated liver disease in two infants with short bowel syndrome using parenteral fish oil: Implications for future management. Pediatrics. 2006;118:e197–e201.

153. Benedetti E, et al. Living related segmental bowel transplantation: From experimental to standardized procedure. Ann Surg. 2006;244:694–699.

154. Fishbein TM. Intestinal transplantation. N Eng J Med. 2009;361:998–1008.

155. Mazariegos GV, et al. Intestine transplantation in the United States, 1999–2008. Am J Transplant. 2010;10:1020–1034.

156. Lopushinsky RA, et al. The optimal timing of intestinal transplantation for children with intestinal failure: A Markov analysis. Ann Surg. 2007;246:1092–1099.

157. Phelan PJ, et al. Renal allograft loss in the first post-operative month: Causes and consequences. Clin Transplant. 2012;26:544–549.

158. Hamed MO, et al. Early graft loss after kidney transplantation: Risk factors and consequences. Am J Transplant. 2015;15:1632–1643.

159. Keller AK, Jorgensen TM, Jespersen B. Identification of risk factors for vascular thrombosis may reduce early renal graft loss: A review of recent literature. J Transplant 2012:793461.

160. Penny MJ, et al. Renal graft thrombosis: A survey of 134 consecutive cases. Transplantation. 1994;58:565–569.

161. Manara A, et al. Donation and transplantation activity in the UK during the COVID-19 lockdown. Lancet. 2020;398(10249):465–466.

162. Götzinger F, et al. COVID-19 in children and adolescents in Europe: A multinational, multicentre cohort study. Lancet. 2020;4(9):653–661.

163. Wei Teoh C, Gaudreault-Tremblay M, Blydt-Hansen T. Management of pediatric kidney transplant patients during the COVID-19 pandemic: Guidance from the Canadian Society of Transplantation Pediatric Group. Can J Kidney Health Dis. 2020;7:1–18.

164. Mallakmir S, et al. Genetic perspectives on paediatric liver transplantation, indications, molecular basis and prognosis. J Gastroenterol Hepatol Res. 2019;4(24):1–7.

165. Kasahara M, et al. Living donor liver transplantation for pediatric patients with metabolic disorders: The Japanese multicenter registry. Pediatr Transplant. 2013;18:6–15.

166. Applegarth DA, Toone JR, Lowry RB. Incidence of inborn errors of metabolism in British Columbia, 1969–1996. Pediatrics. 2000;105:10.

167. Sanderson S, et al. The incidence of inherited metabolic disorders in the West Midlands, UK. Arch Dis Child. 2006;91:896–899.

168. Batshaw ML, et al. A longitudinal study of urea cycle disorders. Mol Genet Metabl. 2014;113:127–130.
169. Piccolo P, Brunetti-Pierri N. Gene therapy for inherited diseases of liver metabolism. Hum Gen Ther. 2015;26:186–192.
170. Spada M, et al. Pediatric liver transplantation. World J Gastroenterol. 2009;15.
171. Adam R, et al. Evolution of indications and results of liver transplantation in Europe: A report from the European Liver Transplant Registry. J Hepatol. 2012;57:675–688.
172. Suchy FJ, et al. *Liver diseases in children.* Cambridge: Cambridge University Press, 2014.
173. Barshes NR, et al. Evaluation and management of patients with propionic acidemia undergoing liver transplantation: A comprehensive review. Pediatr Transplant. 2006;10:773–781.
174. Kabra M. Dietary management of inborn errors of metabolism. Indian J Pediatr. 2002;69:421–426.
175. Murray KF, Carithers RL. AASLD Practice guidelines: Evaluation of the patient for liver transplantation. Hepatol. 2005;41:1407.
176. Burdelsky M, et al. Liver transplantation in children: Long-term outcome and quality of life. Eur J Pediatr. 1999;158(Suppl 2):S34.
177. Jain A, et al. Pediatric liver transplantation: A single center experience spanning 20 years. Transplantation. 2002;73:941.
178. Martin SR, et al. Studies of pediatric liver transplantation 2002: Patient and graft survival and rejection in pediatric recipients of a first liver transplant in the United States and Canada. Pediatr Transplant. 2004;8:273.
179. Kayler LK, et al. Long-term survival after liver transplantation in children with metabolic disorders. Pediatr Transplant. 2002;6:295.
180. Morioka D, et al. Living donor liver transplantation for pediatric patients with inheritable metabolic disorders. Am J Transplant. 2005;5:2754.
181. Mazariegos G, et al. Liver transplantation for pediatric metabolic disease. Mol Genet Metab. 2014;111:418–427.
182. Teckman J, Perlmutter DH. Conceptual advances in the pathogenesis and treatment of childhood metabolic liver disease. Gastroenterol. 1995;108:1263–1279.
183. Toso C, et al. Potential impact of in situ liver splitting on the number of available grafts. Transplantation. 2002;74:222–226.
184. Newstead CG. Assessment of risk of cancer after renal transplantation. Lancet. 1998;351:610–611.
185. Shneider BL. Pediatric liver transplantation in metabolic disease: Clinical decision making. Pediatr Transplant. 2002;6:25.
186. Meyburg J, Hoffmann, GF. Liver transplantation for inborn errors of metabolism. Transplantation. 2005;80(Suppl 1):S135
187. Mckiernan P. Liver transplantation and cell therapies for inborn errors of metabolism. J Inherti Metab Dis. 2013;36:675–680.
188. Faguioli S, et al. Monogenic diseases that can be cured by liver transplantation. J Hepatol. 2013;59:595–612.
189. Brunetti-Pierri N, et al. Acute toxicity after high-dose systemic injection of helper-dependent adenoviral vectors into nonhuman primates. Hum Gene Ther. 2004;15:35–46.
190. Sirrs SM, et al. Barriers to transplantation in adults with inborn errors of metabolism. J Inherit Metab Dis. 2012:139–144.

191. Stevenson T, et al. Long-term outcome following pediatric liver transplantation for metabolic disorders. Pediatr Transplant. 2009;14:268–275.
192. Yuk K, et al. Pediatric liver transplantation for metabolic liver disease: Experience at King's College Hospital. Transplantation. 2009;87:87–93.
193. Baliga P, et al. Post-transplant survival in pediatric fulminant hepatic failure: The SPLIT experience. Liver Transpl. 2004;10:1364.
194. Farmer DG, et al. Liver transplantation for fulminant hepatic failure: Experience with more than 200 patients over a 17-year period. Ann Surg. 2003;237:666.
195. Jaffe R. Liver transplant pathology in pediatric metabolic disorders. Pediatr Dev Pathol. 1998;1:102.
196. Nolkemper D, et al. Long-term results of pre-emptive liver transplantation in primary hyperoxaluria type 1. Pediatr Transplant. 2000;6:25.
197. Rela M, et al. Auxiliary liver transplant for metabolic diseases. Transplant Proc. 1997;29(1–2):444–445.
198. Grossman M, et al. A pilot study of ex vivo gene therapy for homozygous familial hypercholesterolemia. Nat Med.1995;1:1148–1154.
199. Van Malgergem L, et al. Orthotopic liver transplantation from a living-related donor in an infant with a peroxisome biogenesis defect of the infantile Refsum disease type. J Inherit Metab Dis. 2005;28:593–600.
200. Boris-Lawrie K, Temin HM. Recent advances in retrovirus vector technology. Curr Opin Genet Dev. 1993;3:102–109.
201. Miller AD. Retroviral vectors. Curr Top Microbiol Immunol. 1992;158:1–24.
202. Berkner KL. Development of adenovirus vectors for the expression of heterologous genes. Biotechniques. 1988;6:616–629.
203. Berkner KL. Expression of heterologous sequences in adenoviral vectors. Curr Top Microbiol Immunol. 1992;158:39–66.
204. Zabner J, et al. Adenovirus-mediated gene transfer transiently corrects the chloride transport defect in nasal epithelia of patients with cystic fibrosis. Cell. 1993;75:207–216.
205. Geller AI. Herpesviruses: Expression of genes in postmitotic brain cells. Curr Opin Genet Dev. 1993;3:81–85.
206. Kay MA, et al. Expression of human alfa-1-antitrypsin in dogs after autologous transplantation of retroviral transdced hepatocytes. Proc Natl Acad Sci. 1992;89:89–93.
207. Kay MA, et al. Hepatic gene therapy persistent expression of human alfa-antitrypsin in mice after direct gene delivery in vivo. Hum Gene Ther. 1992;3:641–647.
208. Chowdhury JR, et al. Long-term improvement of hypercholesterolemia after ex vivo gene therapy in LDLR-deficient rabbits. Science. 1991;254:1802.
209. Kaleko M, et al. Persistent gene expression after retroviral gene transfer into liver cells in vivo. Hum Gene Ther. 1991;2:27–32.
210. Ferry N, et al. Retroviral-mediated gene transfer into hepatocytes in vivo. Proc Natl Acad Sci USA. 1988:8377–8381.
211. Kay MA, et al. In vivo gene therapy of hemophilia B: Sustained partial correction in factor IX-deficient dogs. Science. 1993;262:117–119.
212. Grossman M, et al. Successful ex vivo gene therapy directed to liver in a patient with familial hypercholesterolaemia Nat Genet. 1994;6:335–341.
213. Stratford-Perricaudet LD, et al. Evaluation of the transfer and expression in mice of an enzyme-encoding gene using a human adenovirus vector. Hum Gene Ther. 1990;3:241–256.
214. Li Q, et al. Assessment of recombinant adeno-viral vectors for hepatic gene therapy. Hum Gene Ther. 1993;4:403–404.

215. Smith T, et al. Adenovirus mediated expression of therapeutic plasma levels of human factor IX in mice. Nat Genet. 1992;1:372–378.
216. Kay MA, et al. In vivo hepatic gene therapy: Complete albeit transient correction of factor IX deficiency in hemophilia B dogs. PNAS. 1994;6:2353–2357.
217. Raper SE, et al. A pilot study of in vivo liver-directed gene transfer with an adenoviral vector in partial ornithine transcarbamylase deficiency. Hum Gene Ther. 2002;13:163–175.
218. Raper SE, et al. Fatal systemic inflammatory response syndrome in a ornithine transcarbamylase deficient patient following adenoviral gene transfer. Mol Genet Metab. 2003;80:148–158.
219. Muruve DA, et al. Adenoviral gene therapy leads to rapid induction of multiple chemokines and acute neutrophil-dependent hepatic injury in vivo. Hum Gene Ther. 1999;10:965–976.
220. Kay M, Savio LC. Gene therapy for metabolic disorders. Rev Trend Genet. 1994;10(7):253–257.
221. Nathwani AC, et al. Adenovirus-associated virus vector-mediated gene transfer in hemophilia B. N Engl J Med. 2011;365:2357–2365.
222. Nathwani AC, et al. Long-term safety and efficacy of factor IX gene therapy in hemophilia B. N Eng J Med. 2014;371:1994–2004.
223. Gonzalez-Aseguinolaza G. Augmenting PBGD expression in the liver as a novel gene therapy for acute intermittent porphyria (AIPgene). Hum Gene Ther Clin Dev. 2014;25:61–63.
224. Eastman SJ, et al. Development of catheter-based procedures for transducing the isolated rabbit liver with plasmid DNA. Hum Gene Ther. 2002;13:2065–2077.
225. Alino SF, et al. Pig liver gene therapy by noninvasive interventionist catheterism. Gene Ther. 2007;14:334–343.
226. Coppoletta JM, Wolbach SB. Body length and organ weights of infants and children: A study of the body length and normal weights of the more important vital organs of the body between birth and twelve years of age. Am J Pathol. 1933;9:55–70.
227. Chandler RJ, et al. Vector design influences hepatic genotoxicity in a murine model. Blood. 2011;117:3311–3319.
228. Donsante A, et al. AAV vector integration sites in mouse hepatocellular carcinoma. Science. 2007;317:477.
229. Yin H, et al. Genome editing with Cas9 in adult mice corrects a disease mutation and phenotype. Nat Biotechnol. 2014;32:551–553.
230. Kasahara M. Living donor liver transplantation for metabolic liver disease. J Pediatr Prac. 2013;76:110–116.
231. McKiernan PKJ. Nitisinone in the treatment of hereditary tyrosinaemia type 1. Drugs. 2006;66:743–750.
232. Masurel-Paulet A, et al. NTBC treatment in tyrosinaemia type 1: Long-term outcome in French patients. J Inherit Metab Dis. 2008;31:81–87.
233. Mohan N, et al. Indications and outcome of liver transplantation in tyrosinaemia type 1. Eur J Pediatr. 1999;158(Suppl 2):S49–S54.
234. Bartlett DC, et al. Early nitisinone treatment reduces the need for liver transplantation in children with tyrosinaemia type 1 and improves post-transplant renal function. J Inherit Metab Dis. 2014;37:745–752.
235. Tuerck J, et al. *Newborn screening follow-up guideline*, 2nd edition. CLSI Document NBS02-A2. Wayne, PA: Clinical & Laboratory Standards Institute, 2013, p. 33.

236. Pierik LJ, et al. Renal function in tyrosinaemia type 1 after liver transplantation: A long-term follow-up. J Inherit Metab Dis. 2005;28:871–876.
237. Bartlett DC, et al. Plasma succinylacetone is persistently raised after liver transplantation in tyrosinaemia type 1. J Inherit Metab Dis. 2013;36:15–20.
238. Matern D, et al. Liver transplantation for glycogen storage disease types I, III, and IV. Eur J Pediat. 1999;158:S43–S48.
239. Maryam M, Pramod M, Michael S. Liver transplantation for inherited metabolic disorders of the liver. Curr Opin Organ Transplant. 2010;15:269–276.
240. Labrune P, et al. Hepatocelluar adenomas in glucogen storage disease type I and III. J Pediatr Gastoenterol Nutr. 1997;24:276–279.
241. Bao Y, et al. Hepatic and neuromuscular forms of glycogen storage disease type IV caused by mutations in the same glycogen-branching enzyme gene. J Clin Invest. 1996;97:941–948.
242. Muraka M, Burlina AB. Liver and liver cell transplantation for glycogen storage disase type IA. Acta Gastroenterol Belg. 2005;48:469–472.
243. Faivre L, et al. Long term outcome of liver transplantation in patients with glycogen storage disease type IA. J Inherit Metab Dis. 1999;22:723–732.
244. LaBrune P. Glycogen storage disease type I: Indications for liver and/or kidney transplantation. Eur J Pediatr. 2002;161:S112–S119.
245. Treem W. Liver transplantation for non-hepatotoxic inborn errors of metabolism. Curr Gastroenterol Rep. 2006;8:213–221.
246. Chiu A, Tsoi NS, Fan ST. Use of the molecular adsorbents recirculating system as a treatment for acute decompensated Wilson disease. Liver Transpl. 2008;14:1512–1516.
247. Medici V, et al. Liver transplantation for Wilson's disease: The burden of neurological and psychiatric disorders. Liver Transpl. 2005;11:1056–1063.
248. Marin C, et al. Liver transplantation in Wilson's disease: Are its indications established? Transplant Proc. 2007;39:2300–2301.
249. Korman JD, et al. Screening for Wilson disease in acute liver failure: A comparison of currently available diagnostic tests. Hepatology. 2008;48:1167–1174.
250. Dhawan A, et al. Wilson's disease in children: 37-year experience and revised King's score for liver transplantation. Liver Transpl. 2005;11:441–448.
251. Sokol RJ, et al. Orthotopic liver transplantation for acute fulminant Wilson disease. J Pediatr. 1985;107:549–552.
252. Yoshitoshi EY, et al. Long-term outcomes for 32 cases of Wilson's disease after living-donor liver transplantation. Transplantation. 2009;87:261–267.
253. Park YK, et al. Auxiliary partial orthotopic living donor liver transplantation in a patient with Wilson's disease: A case report. Transplant Proc. 2008;40:3808–3809.
254. Shilsky ML. Wilson disease: Current status and the future. Biochimie. 2009;91:1278–1281.
255. Kurihara A, et al. Magnetic resonance imaging in late-onset ornithine transcarbamylase deficiency. Brain Dev. 2003;25:40–44.
256. Gropman AL, et al. Diffusion tensor imaging detects areas of abnormal white matter microstructure in patients with partial ornithine transcarbamylase deficiency. Am J Neuroradiol. 2010;31:1719–1723.
257. Prust MJ, Gropman AL, Hauser N. New frontiers in neuroimaging applications to inborn errors of metabolism. Mol Genet Metab. 2011;104(3):195–205.
258. Takanashi J, et al. Distinctly abnormal brain metabolism in late-onset ornithine transcarbamylase deficiency. Neurol. 2002;59:210–214.

259. Gropman AL, et al. 1H MRS allows brain phenotype differentiation in sisters with late onset ornithine transcarbamylase deficiency (OTCD) and discordant clinical presentations. Mol Genet Metab. 2008;94:52–60.

260. Gropman AL, et al. 1H MRS identifies symptomatic and asymptomatic subjects with partial ornithine transcarbamylase deficiency. Mol Genet Metab. 2008;95:21–30.

261. Yorifuji T, et al. X-inactivation pattern in the liver of manifesting female with ornitine transcarbamylase deficiency. Clin Gene. 1998;54:349–353.

262. Wakiya T, et al. Living donor liver transplantation for ornithine transcarbamylase deficiency. Pediatr Transplant. 2011;15:390–395.

263. Inui A, et al. Living related liver transplantation for a ornithine transcarbamylase deficiency. Jap J Pediatr. 1997;101:963–967.

264. Tuchman M. The clinical, biochemical, and molecular spectrum of ornithine transcarbamylase deficiency. J Lab Clin Med. 1992;120:836–850.

265. Ensenaure R, et al. Management and outocme of neonatal-onset ornithine transcarbamylase deficiency following liver transplantation at 60 days of life. Mol Genet Metab. 2005;84:363–366.

266. Moscioni D, et al. Long-term correction of ammonia metabolism and prolonged survival in ornithine transcarbamylase-deficient mice following liver-directed treatment with adeno-associated viral vectors. Mol Ther. 2006;14:25–33.

267. Cunningham SC, et al. Induction and prevention of severe hyperammonemia in the spfash mouse model of ornithine transcarbamylase deficiency using shRNA and rAAV-mediated gene delivery. Mol Ther. 2011;19:854–859.

268. Kok CY, et al. Adeno-associated virus-mediated rescue of neonatal lethality in argninosuccinate synthetase-deficient mice. Mol Ther. 2013;21:1823–1831.

269. Wang L, et al. AAV8-mediated hepatic gene transfer in infant rhesus monkeys (Macaca mulatta). Mol Ther. 2011;19:2012–2020.

270. Leonard JV, Walter J, McKiernan P. The management of organic acidemias: The role of transplantation. J Inherit Metab Dis. 2001;309–314.

271. Blaser S, Feigenbaum, A. A neuroimaging approach to inborn errors of metabolism. Neuroim-Aging Clin N Am. 2004;14:307–329.

272. Radmanesh A, et al. Methylmalonic acidemia: Brain imaging findings in 52 children and a review of the literature. Pediatr Radiol. 2008;38:1054–1061.

273. Brismar J, Ozand PT. CT and MR of the brain in disorders of the propionate and methylmalonate metabolism. Am J Neuroradiol. 1994;15:1459–1473.

274. Lehnert W, et al. Propionic acidemia: Clinical, biochemical and therapeutic aspects: Experience in 30 patients. Eur J Pediatr. 1994;153:S68–S71.

275. Ogier D, Baulny, H. Progress and pitfalls in organic aciduria. Acta Gastroenterol Belg. 2005;48:477–478.

276. Deodato F, et al. Methylmalonic and propionic aciduria. Am J Med Genet C Semin Med Genet. 2006 May 15;142C:104–112 Review.

277. Sato S, et al. Liver transplantation in a patient with propionic acidemia requiring extra corporeal membrane oxygentaion during severe metabolic decompensation. Pediatr Transplant. 2009;88:123–130.

278. Al-Hassnan ZN, et al. The relationship of plasma glutamine to ammonium and of glycine to acid-base balance in propionic acidaemia. J Inherit Metab Dis. 2003;26:89–91.

279. Filipowicz HR, et al. Metabolic changes associated with hyperammonemia in neonatal acute onset prpionic and methylmalonic aciduria. Neonatol. 2010;97:286–290.

280. Filippi L, et al. N-Carbamylglutamate in emergency management of hyperammonemia in neonatal acute onset propionic and methylmalonic aciduria. Neonatology. 2010;97:286–290.

281. Vara R, et al. Liver transplantation for propionic acidemia in children. Liver Transpl. 2011;17:661–667.

282. Yorifuji T, et al. Living-donor liver transplantation for propionic acidaemia. J Inherit Metab Dis. 2004;27:205–210.

283. Fowler B, Leonard JV, Baumgartner MR. Causes of and diagnostic approach to methylmalonic acidurias. J Inherit Metab Dis. 2008;31:350–360.

284. Jansen R, et al. Cloning of full-length methylmalonyl-CoA mutase from a cDNA library using the polymerase chain reaction. Genomics. 1989;4:198–205.

285. Willard HF, Rosenberg LE. Inherited methylmalonyl CoA mutase apoenzyme deficiency in human fibroblasts: Evidence for allelic heterogeneity, genetic compounds, and codominant expression. J Clin Investig. 1980;65:690–698.

286. Brassier A, et al. Renal transplantation in 4 patients with methylmalonic aciduria: A cell therapy for metabolic disease. Mol Genet Metab. 2013:106–110.

287. Schwahn BC, et al. Biochemical efficacy of N-carbamylglutamate in neoantal severe hyperammonaemia due propionic acidaemia. Eur J Pediatr. 2010;169:133–134.

288. Baumgartner MR, et al. Proposed guidelines for the diagnosis and management of methylmalonic and propionic acidemia. Orphanet J Rare Dis. 2014;9:130.

289. Tuchman M, et al. N-Carbamylglutamate markedly enhances ureagenesis in N-acetylglutamate deficiency and propionic acidemia as measured by isotopic incorporatino and blood biomarkers. Pediatr Res. 2008;64:213–217.

290. Hauser NS, et al. Variable dietary management of methylmalonic acidemia: Metabolic and energetic correlations. Am J Clin Nutr. 2011;93:47–56.

291. Lubrano R, et al. Renal transplant in methylmalonic acidemia: Could it be the best option? Report on a case at 10 years and review of the literature. Pediat Nephrol. 2008;22:1209–1214.

292. McGuire PJ, et al. Combined liver-kidney transplant for the management of methylmalonic aciduria: A case report and review of the literature. Mol Genet Metab. 2008:22–29.

293. Cosson MA, et al. Long-Term outcome in methylmalonic aciduia: A series of 30 French patients. Mol Genet Metab. 2009;97:172–178.

294. Burlina AP, et al. Diffusion-weighted imaging in the assessment of neurological damage in patients with methylmalonic aciduria. J Inherit Metab Dis. 2003;26:417–422.

295. Rutledge SL, et al. Tubulointerstitial nephritis in methylmalonic acidemia. Pediatric Nephrol. 1993:1180–1181.

296. Andrews E, et al. Expression of recombinant human methylmalonyl-CoA mutase in primary mut fibroblasts and Saccharomyces cerevisiae. Biochem Med Metabol Biol. 1993;50:135–144.

297. Nagarajan S, Enns GM, Millan MT. Management of methylmalonic acidemia by combined liver-kidney transplantation. J Inherit Metab Dis. 2005;28: 517–524.

298. Van Calcar SC, et al. Renal transplantation in a patient with methylmalonic acidemia. J Inherit Metab Dis. 1998:729–737.

299. Kaplan P, et al. Liver transplantation is not curative for methylmalonic acidopathy caused by methylamalonyl-CoA mutase deficiency. Mol Genet Metab. 2006;88:322–326.

300. Michel SJ, Given CA, Robertson WC. Imaging of the brain, including diffusion-weighted imaging in methylmalonic acidemia. Pediatr Radiol. 2004;34:580–582.

301. Takeuchi M, et al. Magnetic resonance imaging and spectroscopy in a patient with treated methylmalonic acidemia. J Comput Assist Tomogr. 2003;27:547–551.
302. Trinh BC, Melhem ER, Barker, PB. Multi-slice proton MR spectroscopy and diffusion-weighted imaging in methylmalonic acidemia: Report of two cases and review of the literature. Am J Neuroradiol. 2001;22:831–833.
303. Yesildag A, et al. Magnetic resonance imaging and diffusion-weighted imaging in methylmalonic acidemia. Acta Radiol. 2005;46:101–103.
304. Gao Y, et al. Fractional anisotropy for assessment of white matter tracts injury in methylmalonic acidemia. Chin Med J. 2009;122:945–949.
305. Nyhan WL, et al. Progressive neurologic disability in methylmalonic acidemia despite transplantation of the liver. Eur J Pediatr. 2002;161:377–379.
306. Vernon HJ, et al. A detailed analysis of methylmalonic acid kinetics during hemodialysis and after combined liver/kidney transplantation in a patient with mut (0) methylmalonic acidemia. J Inherit Metab Dis. 2014:899–907.
307. Dionisi-Vici C, et al. "Classical" organic acidurias, propionic aciduria, methylmalonic aciduria and isovaleric aciduria: Long-term outcome and effects of expanded newborn screening using tandem mass spectrometry. J Inherit Metab Dis. 2006;29:383–389.
308. Chakrapani A, et al. Metabolic stroke in methylmalonic acidemia 5 years after liver transplantation. J Pediatr. 2002;140:261–263.
309. Ban K, et al. A pediatric patient with classical citrullinemia who underwent living-related partial liver transplanttion. Transplantation. 2001;71:1495.
310. Van der Veere CN, et al. Current therapy for Crigler-Najjar syndrome type 1: Report of a world registry. Hepatology. 1996;24:311–315.
311. Whitington PF, et al. Orthotopic auxiliary liver transplantation for Crigler-Najjar syndrome type 1. Lancet. 1993;342:779–780.
312. Sokal EM, et al. Orthotopic liver transplatation for Crigler-Najjar type I disease in six children. Transplantation. 1995;60:1095–1098.
313. Rela M, et al. Auxiliary partial orthotopic liver transplantation for Crigler-Najjar syndrome type 1. Ann Surg. 1999;229:565–569.
314. Shauer R, et al. Successful liver transplantation of two brothers with Crigler-Najjar syndrome type 1 using a single cadaveric organ. Transplantation. 2002;73: 67–69.
315. Ng VL, et al. Hepatocyte transplantation: Advancing biology and treating children. Clin Liver Dis. 2000;4:929–945.
316. Fox IJ, Roy Chowdhury J, Kaufmann SS. Treatment of the Crigler-Najjar syndrome type I with hepatocyte transplantation. N Engl J Med. 1998;338:1422–1426.
317. Dhawan A, Mitry R, Hughes R. Hepatocyte transplantation for metabolic disorders, experience at Kings College Hospital and review of the literature. Acta Gastroenterol Belg. 2005;68:457–460.
318. Pastore N, et al. Improved efficacy and reduced toxicity by ultrasound-guided intrahepatic injections of helper-dependant adenoviral vector in Gunn rats. Hum Gene Ther Methods. 2013;24:321–327.
319. Chowdhury JR, Kondapalli R, Chowdhury, NR. Gunn rat: A model for inherited deficiency of bilirubin glucuronidation. Adv Vet Sci Comp Med. 1993;37:149–173.
320. Bortolussi G, et al. Rescue of bilirubin induced neonatal lethality in a mouse model of Crigler-Najjar syndrome type 1 by AAV9-mediated gene transfer. FASEB J. 2012;26:1052–1063.
321. Miranda PS, Bosma PJ. Towards liver-directed gene therapy for Crigler-Najjar syndrome. Hum Gene Ther. 2014;25:844–855.

322. Montenegro-Miranda PS, et al. Adeno-associated viral vetor serotype 5 poorly transduces liver in rat models. PLOS One. 2013;8:e82597.
323. Starzl TE, et al. Heart-liver transplantation in a patient with familial hypercholesterolemia. Lancet. 1984;1:1382–1383.
324. Shirahata Y, et al. Living-donor liver transplantation for homozygous familial hypercholesterolemia from a donor with heteroygous hypercholesterolemia. Transpl Int. 2003;16:276–279.
325. Popescu I, et al. Homozygous familial hypercholesterolemia: Specific indication for domino liver transplantation. Transplantation. 2003;76:1345–1350.
326. Popescu I, et al. Domino liver transplant using a graft from a donor with familial hypercholesterolemia: Seven yr follow-up. Clin Transplant. 2009;23:565–570.
327. Liu C, Niu DM, Loong CC, Hsia CY, Tsou MY, Tsai HL, Wei C. Domino liver graft from a patient with homozygous familial hypercholesterolemia. Pediatr Transplant. 2010;14(3):E30–E33. doi:10.1111/j.1399-3046.2009.01133.x.
328. Lebherz C, et al. Gene therapy with novel adeno-associated virus vectors substantially diminishes atherosclerosis in a murine model of familial hypercholesterolemia. J Gene Med. 2004;6:663–672.
329. Kassim SH, et al. Adeno-associated virus serotype 8 gene therapy leads to significant lowering of plasma cholesterol levels in humanized mouse models of homozygous and heterozygous familial hypercholesterolemia. Hum Gene Ther. 2014;24:19–26.
330. Chen SJ, et al. Biodistribution of AAV8 vectors expressing human low-density lipoprotein receptor in a mouse model of homozygous familial hypercholesterolemia. Hum Gene Ther Clin Dev. 2013;24:154–160.
331. Cuchel M, et al. Efficacy and safety of a microsomal triglyceride transfer protein inhibitor in patients with homozygous familial hypercholesterolaemia: A single-arm, open label, phase 3 study. Lancet. 2013;381:40–46.
332. Raal FJ, et al. Mipomersen, an apolipoprotein B synthesis inhibitor, for lowering of LDL cholesterol concentrations in patients with homozygous familial hypercholesterolaemia: A randomised, double-blind, placebo-controlled trial. Lancet. 2010;375:998–1006.
333. Danpure CJ, Jennings PR. Peroisomal alanine: Gloxylate aminotransferase deficiency in primary hyperoxaluria type 1. FEBS Lett. 1986;201:20–24.
334. Mistry J, Danpure CJ, Chalmers RA. Hepatic D-glycerate dehydrogenase and glyoxylate reductase deficiency in primary hyperoxaluria type 2. Biochem Soc Transac. 1988;16:626–627.
335. Varvae BA, et al. Nephrocalcinosis: New insights into mechanisms and consequences. Nephrology Dialysis Transplant. 2009;242030–2035.
336. Hoppe B, et al. The primary hyperoxalurias. Kidney Int. 2009;75:1264–1271.
337. Broyer M, et al. Kidney transplantation in primary oxalosis: Data from the EDTA registry. Nephrology Dialysis Transplant. 1990;5:332–336.
338. Watts RWE, et al. Combined hepatic and renal transplantation in primary hyperoxaluria type 1: Clinical report of 9 cases. Am J Med. 1990;90:179–188.
339. Lieske JC, et al. International registry for primary hyperoxaluria. Am J Nephrol. 2005;25:290–296.
340. Van Woerden CS, et al. Primary hyperoxaluria type 1 in the Netherlands: Prevalence and outcome. Neprhology Dialysis Transplant. 2003;18:273–279.
341. Harambat J, et al. Genotypephenotype correlation in primary hyperoxaluria type 1: The p.Gly170Arg AGXT mutation is associated with a better outcome. Kidney Int. 2010;77:443–449.

342. Leuman EP, et al. New aspects of infantile oxalosis. Pediatric Nephrol. 1987;1:531–535.
343. Ellis SR, et al. Combined liver-kidney transplantation for primary hyperoxaluria type 1 in young children. Nephrology and Dialysis Transplant. 2001;16: 348–354.
344. Bergstralh EJ, et al. Transplantation outcomes in primary hyperoxaluria. Am J Transplant. 2010;10:2493–2501.
345. Jamieson NV. A 20-year experience of combined liver/kidney transplantation for primary hyperoxlaluria (PH1): The European PH1 transplant registry experience 1984–2004. Am J Nephrol. 2005;25:282–289.
346. Astarcioglu I, et al. Primary hyperoxaluria: Simultaneous combined liver and kidney transplantation from a living related donor. Liver Transpl. 2003;9:433.
347. Milliner DS, et al. Primary hyperoxaluria: Results of long-term treatment with orthophosphate and pyridoxine. N Engl J Med. 1994;331:1553–1558.
348. Fargue S, et al. Effect of conservative treatment of the renal outcome of children with primary hyperoxaluria type 1. Kidney Int. 2009;76:767–773.
349. Illies F, et al. Clearance and removal of oxalate in children on intensified dialysis for primary hyperoxaluria type 1. Kidney Int. 2006;70:1642–1648.
350. Latta K, et al. Selection of transplantation procedures and perioperative management in primary hyperoxaluria type 1. Nephrology Dialysis Transplant. 1995; 8:53–57.
351. Monico CG, Milliner D. Combined liver-kidney transplantation and kidney-alone transplantation in primary hyperoxaluria. Liver Transplant. 2001;7:954–963.
352. Scheinman JI, et al. Successful strategies for renal transplantation in primary oxalosis. Kidney Int. 1984;25:804–811.
353. Salido E, et al. Phenotypic correction of a mouse model for primary hyperoxaluria with adeno-associated virus gene transfer. Mol Ther. 2011;19:870–875.
354. Giafi CF, Rumsby, G. Primary hyperoxaluria type 2: Enzymology. J Nephrol. 1998;11:29–31.
355. Marler RA, Montgomery R, Brockmas AW. Diagnosis and treatment of homozygous protein C deficiency. J Pediatr. 1989;114:528–534.
356. Casella J, et al. Successful treatment of homozygous protein C deficiency by hepatic transplantation. Lancet. 1988;1:435–438.
357. Angelis M, et al. En bloc heterotopic auxiliary liver and bilateral renal transplant in a patient with homozygous protein C deficiency. J Pediatr. 2001;138:120–122.
358. Florman S, et al. Multivisceral transplantation for portal hypertension and diffuse mesenteric thrombosis caused by protein C deficiency. Transplantation. 2002;74:406–408.
359. Dhawan A, et al. Hepatocyte transplantation for inherited factor VII deficiency. Transplantation. 2004;78:1812–1814.
360. Dar FS, et al. Outcome of liver transplantation in hereditary hemochromatosis. Transpl Int. 2009;22:717–724.
361. Fenton H, et al. Marked iron in liver explants in the absence of major hereditary hemochromatosis gene defects: A risk factor for cardiac failure. Transplantation. 2009;87:1256–1260.
362. Raichlin E, et al. Combined heart and liver transplantation: A single-center experience. Transplantation. 2009;88:219–225.
363. Adams PC, et al. Is serum hepcidin a causative in hemochromatosis? Novel analysis fro a liver transplant with hemochromatosis. Can J Gastroenterol. 2008;22:851–853.

364. Ismail MK, et al. Transplantationof a liver iwth the C282Y mutation into a recipient heteroygous for H63D results in iron overload. Am J Med Sci. 2009;337: 138–142.

365. Suhr OB, Friman S, Ericzon BG. Early liver transplantation improves familial amyloidotic polyneuropathy patients survival. Amyloid. 2005;12:233–238.

366. Okamoto S, et al. Liver transplantatio for familial amyloidotic polyneuropathy: Impact on Swedish patients survival. Liver Transpl. 2009;15:1229–1235.

367. Niemczyk R, et al. Vitreous amyloidosis in two sisters as the indication of transthyretin-related familial form of sstemic amyloidosis among liver transplantation candidates. Transplant Proc. 2009;41:3085–3087.

368. Stangou AJ, et al. Hereditary fibrinogen A (alpha)-chain amyloidosis: Phenotypic characterization of a systemic disease and the role of liver transplantation. Blood. 2010115:2998–3007.

369. Telles-Correia D, et al. Quality of life following liver transplantation: A comparative study between familial amyloid neuropathy and liver disese patients. BMC Gastroenterol. 2009;9:54.

370. Wahlin S, Harper P, Sardh E, Andersson C, Andersson DE, Ericzon BG. Combined liver and kidney transplantation in acute intermittent porphyria. Transpl Int. 2010;23(6):e18–e21. doi:10.1111/j.1432-2277.2009.01035.x.

371. Strauss KA, Puffenberger EG, Carson VJ. Maple syrup urine disease. In: Adam MP, Feldman J, Mirzaa GM, et al. editors. *Gene reviews*, Seattle, WA: University of Washington, Seattle, 2006, pp. 1993–2023. https://www.ncbi.nlm.nih.gov/books/NBK1319/

372. Strauss KA, et al. Classical maple syrup urine disease and brain development: Principles of managemtn and formula design. Mol Genet Metab. 2010;99:333–345.

373. Nyhan WL, et al. Treatment of the acute crisis in maple syrup urine disease. Arch Pediatr Adolesc Med. 1998;152:593–598.

374. Morton DH, et al. Diagnosis and treatment of maple syrup disease: A study of 36 patients. Pediatrics. 2002;109:999–1008.

375. Strauss KA, Morton DH. Branched-chain ketoacyl dehydrogenase deficiency: Maple syrup disease. Curr Treat Options Neurol. 2003;5:329–341.

376. Jouvet P, et al. Continuous venovenous haemodiafiltration in the acute phase of neonatal maple syrup urine disease. J Inherit Metab Dis. 1997;20:463–472.

377. Yoshino M, et al. Management of acute metabolic decompensation in maple syrup urine disease: A multi-center study. Pediatr Int. 1999;41:132–137.

378. Jouvet P, et al. Combined nutritional support and continuous extracorporeal removal therapy in the severe acute phase of maple syrup urine disease. Intensive Care Med. 2001;27:1798–1806.

379. Ha JS, et al. Maple syrup urine disease encephalopathy: A follow-up study in the acute stage using diffusion-weighted MRI. Pediatr Radiol. 2004;34:163–166.

380. Brismar J, et al. Maple syrup urine disease: findings on CT and MR scans of the brain in 10 infants. AJNR. 1990;11:1219–1228.

381. Parmar H, Sitoh YY, Ho L. Maple syrup urine disease: Diffusion-weighted and diffusion-tensor magnetic resonance imaging findings. J Comput Assist Tomogr. 2004;28:93–97.

382. Jan W, et al. MR diffusion imaging and MR spectroscopy of maple syrup urine disease during acute metabolic decompensation. Neuroradiol. 2003;45:393–399.

383. Heindel W, et al. Proton magnetic resonance spectroscopy reflects metabolic decompensation in maple syrup urine disease. Pediatr Radiol. 1995;25:296–299.

384. Puliyanda DP, et al. Utility of hemodialysis in maple syrup urine disease. Pediatr Nephrol. 2002;17:239–242.

385. Wendel U, et al. Liver transplantation in maple syrup urine disease. Eur J Pediatr. 1999(Suppl 2):S60–S64.

386. Bodner-Leidecker A, et al. Branched chain L-amino acid metabolism in classical maple syrup urine disease after orthotopic liver transplantation. J Inherit Metab Dis. 2000;23:805–818.

387. Strauss KA, et al. Elective liver transplantation for the treatment of classical maple syrup urine disease. Am J Transplant. 2006:557–564.

388. Mazariegos GV, et al. Liver transplantation for classical maple syrup urine disease: Long-term follow-up in 37 patients and comparative united network for organ sharing experience. J Pediatr. 2012;160:116–121.e1.

389. Shellmer DA, et al. Cognitive and adaptative functioning after liver transplantation for maple syrup urine disease: A case sries. Pediatr Transplant. 2011;15(1):58–64.

390. Leonis MA, Balistreri WF. Evaluation and management of end-stage liver disease in children. Gastroenterology. 2008 May;134(6):1741–1751. doi:10.1053/j.gastro.2008.02.029. PMID: 18471551.

391. Bryce CL, Chang CCH, Ren Y, Yabes J, Zenarosa G, Iyer A, et al. Using time-varying models to estimate post-transplant survival in pediatric liver transplant recipients. PLOS One. 2018;13(5):e0198132.

392. Selimoglu MA, Kaya S, Gungor S, Varol FI, Gozukara-Bag HG, Yilmaz S. Infection risk after paediatric liver transplantation. Turk J Pediatr. 2020;62(1):46–52.

393. Nafady-Hego H, Elgendy H, Moghazy WE, Fukuda K, Uemoto S. Pattern of bacterial and fungal infections in the first 3 months after pediatric living donor liver transplantation: An 11-year single-center experience. Liver Transpl. 2011 Aug;17(8):976–984. doi:10.1002/lt.22278. PMID: 21786404.

394. Danziger-Isakov L, Evans HM, Green M, McCulloch M, Michaels MG, Posfay-Barbe KM, et al. Capacity building in pediatric transplant infectious diseases: An international perspective. Pediatr Transplant. 2014;18(8):790–793.

395. Fischer SA, Lu K, Practice ASTIDCo. Screening of donor and recipient in solid organ transplantation. Am J Transplant. 2013;13(Suppl 4):9–21.

396. Verma A, Vimalesvaran S, Dhawan A. Epidemiology, risk factors and outcome due to multidrug resistant organisms in paediatric liver transplant patients in the era of antimicrobial stewardship and screening. Antibiotics (Basel). 2022 Mar 15;11(3):387. doi:10.3390/antibiotics11030387. PMID: 35326850; PMCID: PMC8944546.

397. Fernández J, Prado V, Trebicka J, Amoros A, Gustot T, Wiest R, et al. Multidrug-resistant bacterial infections in patients with decompensated cirrhosis and with acute on chronic liver failure in Europe. J Hepatol. 2019;70:398–411.

398. Errico G, Gagliotti C, Monaco M, Masiero L, Gaibani P, Ambretti S, et al. Colonization and infection due to carbapenemase-producing Enterobacteriaceae in liver and lung transplant recipients and donor-derived transmission: A prospective cohort study conducted in Italy. Clin Microbiol Infect. 2019;25:203–209.

399. Pouch SM, Satlin MJ. Carbapenem-resistant Enterobacteriaceae in special populations: Solid organ transplant recipients, stem cell transplant recipients, and patients with hematologic malignancies. Virulence. 2017;8:391–402.

400. Ferstl PG, Filmann N, Brandt C, Zeuzem S, Hogardt M, Kempf VAJ, et al. The impact of carbapenem resistance on clinical deterioration and mortality in patients with liver disease. Liver Int. 2017;37:1488–1496. [CrossRef]

401. Workowski KA. Centers for Disease Control and Prevention sexually transmitted diseases treatment guidelines. Clin Infect Dis. 2015;61:S759–S762.
402. Verma A, Dhawan A, Wade JJ, Lim WH, Ruiz G, Price JF, et al. Mycobacterium tuberculosis infection in pediatric liver transplant recipients. Pediatr Infect Dis J. 2000;19(7):625–630.
403. Jafri SM, Singal AG, Kaul D, Fontana RJ. Detection and management of latent tuberculosis in liver transplant patients. Liver Transplant. 2011;17:306–314.
404. Fábrega E, Sampedro B, Cabezas J, Casafont F, Mieses MÁ, Moraleja I, et al. Chemoprophylaxis with isoniazid in liver transplant recipients. Liver Transplant. 2012;18:1110–1117.
405. Verma A, Wade JJ. Immunization issues before and after solid organ transplantation in children. Pediatr Transplant. 2006;10(5):536–548.
406. Feldman AG, Kempe A, Beaty BL, Sundaram SS, Studies of Pediatric Liver Transplantation (SPLIT) Research Group. Immunization practices among pediatric transplant hepatologists. Pediatr Transplant. 2016;20(8):1038–1044. doi:10.1111/petr.12765.
407. Chong PP, Avery RK. A comprehensive review of immunization practices in solid organ transplant and hematopoietic stem cell transplant recipients. Clin Ther. 2017;39(8):1581–1598.
408. Rubin LG, Levin MJ, Ljungman P, Davies EG, Avery R, Tomblyn M, et al. 2013 IDSA clinical practice guideline for vaccination of the immunocompromised host. Clin Infect Dis. 2014;58(3):309–318.
409. Danziger-Isakov L, Kumar D, AST ID Community of Practice. Vaccination of solid organ transplant candidates and recipients: Guidelines from the American Society of Transplantation Infectious Diseases Community of Practice. Clin Transplant. 2019;33:e13563.
410. Suresh S, Upton J, Green M, Pham-Huy A, Posfay-Barbe KM, Michaels MG, Top KA, Avitzur Y, Burton C, Chong PP, Danziger-Isakov L, Dipchand AI, Hébert D, Kumar D, Morris SK, Nalli N, Ng VL, Nicholas SK, Robinson JL, Solomon M, Tapiero B, Verma A, Walter JE, Allen UD. Live vaccines after pediatric solid organ transplant: Proceedings of a consensus meeting, 2018. Pediatr Transplant. 2019 Nov;23(7):e13571. doi:10.1111/petr.13571. Epub 2019 Sep 9. PMID: 31497926.
411. Kemme S, Kohut TJ, Boster JM, Diamond T, Rand EB, Feldman AG. Live vaccines in pediatric liver transplant recipients: "To give or not to give". Clin Liver Dis (Hoboken). 2021 Oct 27;18(4):204–210. doi:10.1002/cld.1123. PMID: 34745579; PMCID: PMC8549714.
412. Sun HY, Cacciarelli TV, Singh N. Identifying a targeted population at high risk for infections after liver transplantation in the MELD era. Clin Transplant. 2011;25:420–425. [CrossRef]
413. Hauschild J, Bruns N, Lainka E, Dohna-Schwake C. A European international multicentre survey on the current practice of perioperative antibiotic prophylaxis for paediatric liver transplantations. Antibiotics (Basel). 2023 Feb 1;12(2):292. doi:10.3390/antibiotics12020292. PMID: 36830202; PMCID: PMC9952614.
414. Dohna Schwake C, Guiddir T, Cuzon G, Benissa MR, Dubois C, Miatello J, et al. Bacterial infections in children after liver transplantation: A single-center surveillance study of 345 consecutive transplantations. Transpl Infect Dis. 2020;22(1):e13208.
415. Pouladfar G, Jafarpour Z, Malek Hosseini SA, Firoozifar M, Rasekh R, Khosravi-fard L. Bacterial infections in pediatric patients during early post liver transplant period: A prospective study in Iran. Transpl Infect Dis. 2019;21(1):e13001.

416. Shoji K, Funaki T, Kasahara M, Sakamoto S, Fukuda A, Vaida F, et al. Risk factors for bloodstream infection after living-donor liver transplantation in children. Pediatr Infect Dis J. 2015;34(10):1063–1068.

417. Møller DL, Sørensen SS, Wareham NE, Rezahosseini O, Knudsen AD, Knudsen JD, Rasmussen A, Nielsen SD. Bacterial and fungal bloodstream infections in pediatric liver and kidney transplant recipients. BMC Infect Dis. 2021 Jun 8;21(1):541. doi:10.1186/s12879-021-06224-2. PMID: 34103013; PMCID: PMC8188646.

418. Hollenbeak CS, Alfrey EJ, Sheridan K, Burger TL, Dillon PW. Surgical site infections following pediatric liver transplantation: Risks and costs. Transpl Infect Dis. 2003;5:72–78. doi:10.1034/j.1399-3062.2003.00013.x.

419. Abdullatif H, Dhawan A, Verma A. Epidemiology and risk factors for viral infections in pediatric liver transplant recipients and impact on outcome. Viruses. 2023 Apr 26;15(5):1059. doi:10.3390/v15051059. PMID: 37243144; PMCID: PMC10222744.

420. Li C, Wen TF, Mi K, Wang C, Yan LN, Li B. Analysis of infections in the first 3-month after living donor liver transplantation. World J Gastroenterol. 2012;18:1975–1980. [CrossRef]

421. Fishman JA. Infection in organ transplantation. Am J Transplant. 2017;17:856–879.

422. Rubin RH. The direct and indirect effects of infection in liver transplantation: Pathogenesis, impact, and clinical management. Curr Clin Top Infect Dis. 2002;22:125–154.

423. Alcamo AM, Alessi LJ, Vehovic SN, Bansal N, Bond GJ, Carcillo JA, Green M, Michaels MG., Aneja RK. Severe sepsis in pediatric liver transplant patients: The emergence of multidrug-resistant organisms. Pediatr Crit Care Med. 2019;20:e326–e332. doi:10.1097/PCC.0000000000001983.

424. Phichaphop C, Apiwattanakul N, Techasaensiri C, Lertudomphonwanit C, Treepongkaruna S, Thirapattaraphan C, Boonsathorn S. High prevalence of multidrug-resistant gram-negative bacterial infection following pediatric liver transplantation. Medicine. 2020;99:e23169. doi:10.1097/MD.0000000000023169.

425. Alcamo AM, Trivedi MK, Dulabon C, Horvat CM, Bond GJ, Carcillo JA, Green M, Michaels MG, Aneja RK. Multidrug-resistant organisms: A significant cause of severe sepsis in pediatric intestinal and multi-visceral transplantation. Am J Transplant. 2022 Jan;22(1):122–129. doi:10.1111/ajt.16756. Epub 2021 Jul 28. PMID: 34245113; PMCID: PMC8720054.

426. Sood G, Perl TM. Outbreaks in health care settings. Infect Dis Clin North Am. 2016;30(3):661–687.

427. Verma A, Dhawan A, Philpott-Howard J, Rela M, Heaton N, Vergani GM, et al. Glycopeptide-resistant enterococcus faecium infections in paediatric liver transplant recipients: Safety and clinical efficacy of quinupristin/dalfopristin. J Antimicrob Chemother. 2001;47(1):105–108.

428. Hand J, Patel G. Multidrug-resistant organisms in liver transplant: Mitigating risk and managing infections. Liver Transpl. 2016;22(8):1143–1153.

429. Macesic N, Gomez-Simmonds A, Sullivan SB, Giddins MJ, Ferguson SA, Korakavi G, et al. Genomic surveillance reveals diversity of multidrug-resistant organism colonization and infection: A prospective cohort study in liver transplant recipients. Clin Infect Dis. 2018;67(6):905–912.

430. Ashkenazi-Hoffnung L, Mozer-Glassberg Y, Bilavsky E, Yassin R, Shamir R, Amir J. Children post liver transplantation hospitalized with fever are at a high risk for bacterial infections. Transpl Infect Dis. 2016;18(3):333–340.

431. Sudan DL, Shaw Jr BW, Langnas AN. Causes of late mortality in pediatric liver transplant recipients. Ann Surg. 1998;227(2):289–295.

432. Tascini C, Sbrana F, Flammini S, Tagliaferri E, Arena F, Leonildi A, et al. Oral gentamicin gut decontamination for prevention of KPC-producing K pneumoniae infections: Relevance of concomitant systemic antibiotic therapy. Antimicrob Agents Chemother. 2014;58:1972–1976.

433. Freire MP, Oshiro IC, Pierrotti LC, Bonazzi PR, de Oliveira LM, Song AT, et al. Carbapenem-resistant enterobacteriaceae acquired before liver transplantation: Impact on recipient outcomes. Transplantation. 2017;101(4):811–820.

434. Verma A, Wade JJ, Cheeseman P, Samaroo B, Rela M, Heaton ND, et al. Risk factors for fungal infection in paediatric liver transplant recipients. Pediatr Transplant. 2005;9(2):220–225.

435. Lehrnbecher T, Robinson PD, Fisher BT, Castagnola E, Groll AH, Steinbach WJ, et al. Galactomannan, beta-D-glucan, and polymerase chain reaction-based assays for the diagnosis of invasive fungal disease in pediatric cancer and hematopoietic stem cell transplantation: A systematic review and meta-analysis. Clin Infect Dis. 2016;63(10):1340–1348.

436. Aslam S, Rotstein C, AST Infectious Disease Community of Practice. Candida infections in solid organ transplantation: Guidelines from the American Society of Transplantation Infectious Diseases Community of Practice. Clin Transplant. 2019;33. [CrossRef]

437. Verma A, Weigel KS, Dexter SYK, Dhawan A. Evolution in the management of invasive fungal infections in liver transplant recipients. OBM Transplant. 2018;2. doi:10.21926/obm.transplant.1802009.

438. Verma A, Auzinger G, Kantecki M, Campling J, Spurden D, Percival F, et al. Safety and efficacy of anidulafungin for fungal infection in patients with liver dysfunction or multiorgan failure. Open Forum Infect Dis. 2016;4:ofw241.

439. Patterson TF, Thompson GR III, Denning DW, Fishman JA, Hadley S, Herbrecht R, Kontoyiannis DP, Marr KA, Morrison VA, Nguyen MH, Segal BH, Steinbach WJ, Stevens DA, Walsh TJ, Wingard JR, Young JA, Bennett JE. Practice guidelines for the diagnosis and management of aspergillosis: 2016 update by the Infectious Diseases Society of America. Clin Infect Dis. 2016 Aug 15;63(4):e1–e60. doi:10.1093/cid/ciw326. Epub 2016 Jun 29. PMID: 27365388; PMCID: PMC4967602.

440. Cherian T, Giakoustidis A, Yokoyama S, O'Grady J, Rela M, Wendon J, et al. Treatment of refractory cerebral aspergillosis in a liver transplant recipient with voriconazole: Case report and review of the literature. Exp Clin Transplant. 2012;10:482–486.

441. Onishi A, Sugiyama D, Kogata Y, Saegusa J, Sugimoto T, Kawano S, et al. Diagnostic accuracy of serum 1,3-beta-D-glucan for *Pneumocystis jiroveci* pneumonia, invasive candidiasis, and invasive aspergillosis: Systematic review and meta-analysis. J Clin Microbiol. 2012;50:7–15.

442. Onpoaree N, Sanpavat A, Sintusek P. Cytomegalovirus infection in liver-transplanted children. World J Hepatol. 2022 Feb 27;14(2):338–353. doi:10.4254/wjh.v14.i2.338. PMID: 35317177; PMCID: PMC8891677.

443. Verma A, Palaniswamy K, Cremonini G, Heaton N, Dhawan A. Late cytomegalovirus infection in children: High incidence of allograft rejection and hepatitis in donor negative and seropositive liver transplant recipients. Pediatr Transplant. 2017 May;21(3). doi:10.1111/petr.12879. Epub 2017 Jan 30. PMID: 28134467.

444. Pappo A, Peled O, Berkovitch M, Bilavsky E, Rom E, Amir J, Krause I, Yarden-Bilavsky H, Scheuerman O, Ashkenazi-Hoffnung L. Efficacy and safety of a weight-based dosing regimen of valganciclovir for cytomegalovirus prophylaxis in pediatric solid-organ transplant recipients. Transplantation. 2019;103:1730–1735.

445. Green M, Michaels M. Epstein-Barr virus infection and post transplant lymphoproliferative disorder. Am J Transplant. 2013;13:41–45. [CrossRef]

446. Okamoto T, Okajima H, Uebayashi EY, Ogawa E, Yamada Y, Umeda K, Hiramatsu H, Hatano E. Management of Epstein-Barr virus infection and post-transplant lymphoproliferative disorder in pediatric liver transplantation. J Clin Med. 2022 Apr 13;11(8):2166. doi:10.3390/jcm11082166. PMID: 35456259; PMCID: PMC9031649.

447. Allen UD, Preiksaitis JK, AST Community of Practice. Post-transplant lymphoproliferative disorders, Epstein-Barr virus infection, and disease in solid organ transplantation: Guidelines from the American Society of Transplantation Infectious Diseases Community of Practice. Clin Transplant. 2019;33(9):e13652. PMID: 31230381.

448. Chang YC, Young RR, Mavis AM, Chambers ET, Kirmani S, Kelly MS, Kalu IC, Smith MJ, Lugo DJ. Epstein-Barr Virus DNAemia and post-transplant lymphoproliferative disorder in pediatric solid organ transplant recipients. PLOS One. 2022 Oct 18;17(10):e0269766. doi:10.1371/journal.pone.0269766. PMID: 36256635; PMCID: PMC9578615.

Index

Note: Page numbers in *italics* indicate a figure and page numbers in **bold** indicate a table on the corresponding page.

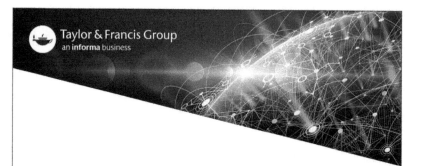

Milton Keynes UK
Ingram Content Group UK Ltd.
UKHW022042141024
449569UK00022B/787

9 781032 371320